The Sistahs' Rules

The Sistahs' Rules

Secrets for Meeting, Getting, and
Keeping a Good Black Man

Denene Millner

Quill
William Morrow
New York

It is the policy of William Morrow and Company, Inc., and its imprints and affiliates, recognizing the importance of preserving what has been written, to print the books we publish on acid-free paper, and we exert our best efforts to that end.

Millner, Denene.
    The sistahs' rules : secrets for meeting, getting, and keeping a good black man / Denene Millner.
        p.   cm.
    ISBN 0-688-15689-4
    1. Man-woman relationships.   2. Afro-American men.   I. Title.
HQ801.M575   1997
646.7'7—dc21   97-21792
                                                                                      CIP

Printed in the United States of America

First Edition

10

BOOK DESIGN BY RENATO STANISIC

Dedication

For Daddy, whose love, strength, and will
exemplify the term "good black man."
For Mommy, whose love, strength, and will
helped her recognize one when she saw one.
And for Nick, who helped me reach my level.

Contents

Introduction: The Sistahs' Rules Is All About You
xiii

How to Meet a Good Black Man
1

Rule # 1: Celebrate the Power of the Booty
3

Rule # 2: Get a Life
8

Rule # 3: Hook It Up, Girl!
13

Rule # 4: Get That Wish List in Order
19

Rule # 5: Get Out of His Wallet
24

Rule # 6: Use Your Heart and Not Your Eyes
30

Rule # 7: Use What You Got to Get What You Want
34

Rule # 8: Go Get Him, Girl!
39

Rule # 9: If He Gives You a Pager Number Instead of the
Digits, Dump His Butt (And Other Recognizable Signals
That Indicate You Need to Kick Him to the Curb)
44

Rule # 10: If He Sends You Flowers Just Because,
He Could Be a Keeper (And Other Recognizable Signals
That Indicate He's Your Potential Brother Mr. Right)
49

Rule # 11: Call the Brother, Date the Brother
54

How to Get a Good Black Man
59

Rule # 12: How to Work It on Your First Few Dates,
Before You Get to Doing the Nasty
61

Rule # 13: No Swerving on the First Date
66

Rule # 14: Blow His Mind
70

Rule # 15: The Way to a Man's Heart Is Through
a Great Plate of Greens
74

Rule # 16: Grab a Playbook and Learn
Michael Jordan's Moves
79

Rule # **17**: Don't Get All Worked Up Because He
Forgot Your Birthday or Buys You Cheap Gifts
85

Rule # **18**: Shield Your Building from the Blaze
90

Rule # **19**: After You Get Your Swerve On, Leave Him
94

Rule # **20**: How to Determine He's into You and Not
Just the Nookie
98

Rule # **21**: Don't Compare Him to Your Last Man
102

Rule # **22**: Girlfriends Are Everything, but
They Don't Know It All
106

Rule # **23**: Be His Homie
114

Rule # **24**: Get to Know His Mama, Get to Know Him
119

Rule # **25**: Don't Mention the "M" Word for at Least
Twelve Months
127

Rule # **26**: Give Him the Option of Commitment
133

How to Keep a Good Black Man
139

Rule # 27: Give Him Three Months After He Commits to
Tie Up Loose Ends
141

Rule # 28: Make Your Past Relationships
Official Black History
146

Rule # 29: You Don't Wear a Cape, So Don't
Try to Be Superwoman
151

Rule # 30: Never Ask a Question You Don't Want
the Answer To
155

Rule # 31: Channel the Bitch Sessions, Keep a Man
161

Rule # 32: Be His Lover, Not His Mother
167

Rule # 33: Getting to Know His Mother and Sisters Goes
a Long Way
174

Rule # 34: Shack Up
179

Rule # 35: Share the Household Responsibilities
185

More Sistahs' Rules
191

Rule # 36: Leave Her Man Alone
193

Rule # 37: If He Wants Out or He's Not Acting Right,
Show Him the Door
198

Rule # 38: So You Got Dissed, Huh? Get Over It!
203

Rule # 39: Rules for High School Sistahs
207

Rule # 40: Rules for College Sistahs
212

Acknowledgments
217

Introduction

The Sistahs' Rules Is All About You

The Rules?

Puh-leeze, girl. Any real black woman can tell you that when it comes to African-American men, the oft-celebrated *Rules* is about as good as a pile of Monopoly money in Macy's.

Useless.

Try waiting for a brother to call you, when you rarely return his phone calls.

Try playing coy and mysterious with him on your first date.

Try sitting back and giving him all the power to make all the decisions in your relationship.

You'd be better off acquainting yourself with the Friday evening television lineup, because you'll be spending an awful lot of time on the sofa in front of the TV—remote in one hand, corn chips in the other—wasting quality weekend time with yourself, by yourself. No eligible black man would play the game by *those* rules—and you sistahs know this.

So a growing chorus of you continue to shout the same question from the rooftops: Where are the good black men and how can I get one?

Of course, lament over the shortage of "good ones" is universal—and the popularity of *The Rules* proves the topic certainly stretches across all age, ethnic, and racial lines.

But nobody seems to have the knack for vocalizing loneliness better than us sistahs—as witnessed by the *Waiting to Exhale* sistah-girlfriend clutches on black relationships, and the phenomenal sales of black relationship books.

The problem is that we've all too often held our potential mates up against the Knight in Shining Armor standards adopted by some of our white contemporaries—a fantasy wish list that's sentencing us sistahs to the singles-only line.

I have to admit, it's pretty difficult to hold black men to different standards, particularly when we're constantly barraged with statistics that portray the "endangered black male" as more likely than not to be uneducated, unemployed, with a prison record and a history of either using or selling drugs, gay, married, dead, or otherwise socially unavailable.

And we can't ignore the growing numbers of upwardly mobile black men bypassing their female counterparts, only to take up with white ones—or those who, recognizing they're at the top of the most eligible bachelors' list, are forsaking marriage for the swinging singles life.

We've even got some brothers out there who say they can afford to be "picky" and "playas"—that is, date a host of women at the same time—because society's taught them that their education, career title, salary, and 401(k) plan place them squarely in the "in serious demand" category. And they'll readily play the game, too—put on their running shoes to get to Nia if Roslyn doesn't give them what they want.

No, sis—the games may work on the other men, but not on our men.

It's enough to make us sistahs—who always dreamed of sharing our lives with men who have just as much or more than we have—pondering whether we'll be living out those white-picket-fence dreams *without* the dashing black prince in the shiny white Benz.

We're tired of chasing them, tired of trying to get them to notice us, tired of hearing our clocks ticking and nobody setting off the alarm—just tired, tired, tired.

Well, I'm telling you that there are good black men out there—ones who are ready, willing, and able to make you happy if you give them a chance and you work it just right. It's going to take a little bit more running, sistah—but this is for that good race, the one that will have him standing up and cheering you front row and center on your very own sideline. All you have to do is follow the Sistahs' Rules.

I'll tell you how to spot out a "good" one and how to tell

when he's a loser, where to meet him, how to approach him, and how to act on the first date. I'll clue you in on how to tell if he seriously likes you, when to sleep with him, and how to tell if he likes you or the sex.

I'll share with you all my secrets for capturing his heart.

Now, there's going to be some sistahs who think these rules are over the top—that there's no need to practice Rule # 5, in which I tell you to stop looking for men with money, or Rules # 15, 16 and 17, where I tell you to cook for him, learn about sports, and get over the fact that he didn't buy you a gift. I've already had sistahs bending my ear, complaining that we black women are just too darn preoccupied with getting the ring and authors like me are spending entirely too much time telling women to bend over backward for those "sorry-ass men."

"Why do we continue to fill ourselves with this nonsense?" one of my colleagues fumed when she heard about Sistahs' Rules. "When are we going to learn that we don't need men? And why can't a black man write a book about how to please *us*?"

Well, I'll tell you why. Relationships are important to us; we look forward to having companions and sharing the most intimate part of our lives with significant others. We want that stable relationship—that "forever" stability like the kind my parents and in-laws have. We want to raise healthy kids in a safe environment with a loving mate. We want men—not in front of us, not behind us, but beside us—to accompany us through this trip called life.

And we don't mind asking someone to help us find him.

Anyone who doesn't have one and claims she doesn't need one is either fooling herself or plain not interested in men.

Now, I wouldn't mind picking up a book by a black man that explains detail for detail what brothers need to do to please my behind. But I think it's pretty pointless to sit around holding your breath, being lonely and bitter, while you wait for the brothers to come around. I wouldn't waste my time doing it.

Neither should you.

Read Sistahs' Rules. Memorize Sistahs' Rules. Use Sistahs' Rules. Then prepare yourself for a life filled with happiness as your Brother Mr. Right comes strolling into your life. You won't know how you survived this long without them—or him.

The Sistahs' Rules

How
TO MEET
A GOOD
BLACK MAN

Celebrate the Power of the Booty

Be proud to be *you*.

Don't ever let your quest to attract a black man drive you to try to squeeze your thick nose, your kinky hair, and that round bottom into white folks' beauty standards—because they'll never, ever fit, no matter how hard you push and shove.

It's pretty obvious, after all, that God didn't make that Cindy Crawford mold with a sistah in mind.

But we spend an awful lot of time trying to get into it, don't we? We'll give our last dollar for advice on how to flatten our butts, how to get rid of those "thunder thighs," how to slather on the best relaxers to get our hair the straightest it can possibly get—and then beat the hell out of ourselves when Cindy fails to magically appear in our mirrors.

Get over it, girls. We are no more able to transform ourselves into bone-thin, blond-haired, blue-eyed beauties than she's able to transform herself into a dreadlocked chocolate honey with dark brown eyes and an hourglass figure that'd make the Commodores leave Ms. "Brick House."

Besides, most black men would rather fatten up that bony-butt Cindy with a big plate of greens and cornbread than date her, because for them, to be too thin is a sin.

The simple fact is that a good black man will like you just the way you are—big butt, thick thighs, blackness, and all. The sooner you accept and appreciate your unique beauty, the sooner it will be obvious that you are proud of being you. The sooner you carry yourself as if you are the fiercest creature to walk this earth since Foxy Brown, the sooner will come a black man who thinks the same about you.

Now, it took me awhile to get a grasp of this one. We come from a culture where, just a short time ago, our very own people accepted and enforced that saying "If you look white, you're all right, but if you're black, get back"—and I, like a lot of our folks, took it to heart.

A few years ago, you'd have never caught me in red, because I was always taught that dark-skinned people like me weren't supposed to wear bright colors. They'd just make me look "blacker," and Lord knows I didn't want that.

And at one point in my life, you'd have had to hold a gun to my head to get me in the pool or to sit out in the sun—because Ms. Denene didn't want her melanin to go into overdrive and make her skin any darker than it already was, and she certainly didn't want her firmly pressed hair to get "nappy."

The most disturbing thing I did to myself, though, was to regard my big butt as a curse. When I was younger, those slick Jordache jeans were the rage, and you had to be bone thin to get in them. Naturally, my butt was made for Jordache like a circle was meant to fit a square peg. So I did just about everything I could to try to make it just go away, including crawling on the floor with my butt backward to try to lose the inches. It was a stupid and downright fruitless endeavor, I realized, after I stopped to think about it for a minute. But that didn't stop me from hiding my butt under baggy pants and sweaters so as not to call attention to it.

Then a friend of mine convinced me to model in a fashion show at the college where I studied. I told her I was cool with wearing whatever, but "please, no tight stuff." She said, "No problem."

She lied.

When we got to that auditorium and the seats filled up and everyone in the dressing room was shrouded in a hail of makeup brushes and stilettos and hot combs and curling irons, girlfriend flipped on me: She pulled out this tight, short, little red-leather number. "You're the only one who can fit it," she said, shrugging. Its saving grace was that it had a matching red jacket cut long enough to cover most of my butt and hips. That I was wearing it, though, was disturbing the basketball team, which had made it known they were sitting in the front rows to see bodies, not clothes. As I walked down one catwalk and across to another, a few yelled, "Take off the jacket!" Embarrassed, I ignored them—until they started chanting it.

So I took it off.

The guys went nuts. One proposed. A few of them followed me across the campus like a bunch of drooling puppies for the next semester.

It took all of that for me to recognize there's, as comedienne Phyllis Stickney once so poetically put it, "power in the booty." She wasn't lying when she said black men will do anything—anything—to please a woman with a big butt, and we, as black women, need to take advantage of that.

Of course, nothing is ever that simple; black men will not just fall to their knees at the mere sight of you and your glorious booty. But I can testify today that the moment I started appreciating my body and my skin and just plain being black is the moment I started attracting black men. See, a woman who is sexy and proud and confident in herself is that much more attractive and sexy to a brother; she's magnetic, and he is drawn to her because she looks like she has it all together—even if everyone else just doesn't get it. Your assuredness will let him know he doesn't have to compliment you constantly—though he will feel compelled to do so because *you are bad*.

The fact is that we are the shades of almond and Hershey's

special dark chocolate, coffee with three splashes of cream, and milk with four drops of vanilla extract. We wear our hair relaxed and pincurled, pressed, in dreads, cornrowed and in short afros. We are tall and short, thick and not-so-thick, curvy and slim. We are, to borrow a line from the seventies Black Power Movement, "black and beautiful"—no matter the shade and shape— and we need to celebrate that, rather than insecurely trying to jibe with what's on the front cover of the latest magazine.

If he's looking for Cindy, let him chase her down on the catwalk. The other brothers, the ones who appreciate a beautiful woman secure with her blackness, will be too busy hunting you down to be bothered with her anyway.

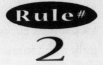

Get a Life

This sistah I used to hang with back in the day had a really simple formula for weeding out the black men she thought weren't good enough for her: If he even looked like he couldn't provide her with what she was "accustomed to"—the house, the car, the pool, the clothes, and a certain lifestyle—then he need not apply.

What was most humorous about her ultimatums was that she hadn't a clue what it was like to have those things. What sistah-girl was "accustomed to" was living with her mother in the projects, making seven dollars an hour as a glorified secretary at a community center right around the corner from where she lived, and barely getting by. She didn't have a car, she never saw any kind of pool other than the public one the next town over, and her clothes—well, that was a whole 'nother story altogether.

Not that there's anything wrong with projects and seven dollars an hour and community centers and secretaries; it's honorable living and honorable work if you can find it these days. What I found most ironic about my girl, though, was that she truly expected a complete stranger to give her all the material wealth and good living she ever dreamed of—yet she didn't respect herself enough to get those things on her own. If I were a self-respecting black man with a decent amount of loot and the ability to let my lady live comfortably, I wouldn't give her the time of day, either.

And why should he?

The brother who worked hard for that degree and busted his ass for that title isn't about to siphon off his sweets to a sistah who can't bring some of her own goods to the table—and I can't say I blame him. They can recognize golddiggers coming a mile away.

We sistahs were raised better than that, anyway. Our mamas taught us to be self-sufficient, strong and independent—to work hard for what we want, because nobody else is going to do it for us. Inherent in that lesson was that we should never, ever sit around waiting for some man to make us happy with material goods, because if we couldn't find a man who could do it, we'd be setting ourselves up for a serious fall. It would be nice if he could provide what we'd like to think we could get "accustomed to," they told us—but don't count on it.

It's a pearl of wisdom to live by.

If you don't like living in the projects, you're feeling like your seven-dollar-an-hour job is a dead end, and there are a lot more things you could stand to have in your life, change it *yourself.* Maya Angelou wrote in her book *Wouldn't Take Nothing for My Journey Now* that it's a strong woman who recognizes when it's time to change paths:

"Each of us has the right and the responsibility to assess the roads which lie ahead, and those over which we have traveled, and if the future road looms ominous or unpromising, and the roads back uninviting, then we need to gather our resolve and, carrying only the necessary baggage, step off that road into another direction. If the new choice is also unpalatable, without embarrassment, we must be ready to change that as well."

A Sistahs' Rules girl knows right off that stepping from that road into another direction is a decision that she has to make for herself, and a mission that she has to carry out herself. She doesn't sit around waiting to get rich by marrying some man. She goes to college. She gets her own career, makes her own piles of money, buys her own homes and cars and clothes— creates her own fame.

And if she finds a man who can add to those things she's gotten for herself, fine. If he comes to the table empty-handed but with a warm heart and a generous spirit, that's fine too—because you will have already gotten what you're "accustomed to."

I always knew this, but it hit home recently while I was out working on a story about the wives of the Knicks, New York's professional basketball team. I walked into Madison Square Garden convinced that these ladies were going to be nothing more than a bunch of pretty girls who got rich and launched themselves into the celebrity spotlight with a single stroll down the aisle—that they would have never been capable of being the fly girls they were if they weren't married to some of the country's richest black men.

To the contrary, these women were indeed no fools. Charlie Ward's wife, Tonja, is an attorney, who, when I interviewed her, was trying to decide if she was going to join a law firm or if she was going to open her own practice. Deborah Williams, wife of Herb Williams, is a psychologist who, between consulting jobs with the NBA and New York area hospitals, is the proud designer of her own clothing line—a longtime dream of this fashion plate. Allan Houston's wife, Tamara, was in the midst of deciding if she was going to go to law school or if she would take a detour first and go for her master's in business.

These women were sitting at the table talking about how they could further their careers—not how they could live off their husbands' money. By the time I left there, I felt guilty for assuming they were taking great pleasure in simply basking in their husbands' spotlights; clearly, they all would have done well for themselves even if they hadn't married into the NBA.

I have another girlfriend who wishes she had thought of that before she married a professional football player. She went to college, but used that valuable time chasing after this player instead of making sure she was preparing herself for a career in marketing, her major. When she graduated, she married him— and immediately dropped all plans to pursue a job in her field of study. Ten years later, his career was over, he was sleeping around, dabbling in drugs, and looking for a pen so that she could sign the divorce papers—and coming up with every excuse in the book for why he couldn't pay child support. Now she's got three kids, a house she won in the divorce settlement but can't pay for, and a coulda-woulda-shoulda rap about how if she hadn't married that trifling man she would have had a nice career and wouldn't be worried about where the money for the next mortgage payment was coming from.

She's thinking about going back to school to brush up on those marketing skills. There's good money to be made there.

Now she just needs to figure out what to do with the kids.

Hey—at least she's following Maya Angelou's advice: It's never too late to change paths.

But you should make sure that you put yourself on the right one early—and stay away from the one that dictates you depend on him for what you're "accustomed to."

Like my friend, you just might get too accustomed to it.

Hook It Up, Girl!

It certainly doesn't take a rocket scientist to figure out that a chick who would dare be seen in
public looking tore up from the floor up
wouldn't rate a second look from a brother.

The obvious explanation for this is as clear as
the sky is blue: No black man wants, as my daddy
used to call it, a "ragglely" woman. You know the
kind: the one who more often than not goes out
the house looking like she crawled out of bed not
more than five minutes ago, fell into her outfit,
picked up the comb but barely used it, and stum-
bled out the door.

Hated it! How is your next-door neighbor—

the one that looks just like Denzel—going to notice you if you consistently look like who hit it and ran?

Check it out: The way you look is the first thing he's going to notice—and I don't have to tell you how important first impressions are. This is your chance to let it be known that you care about yourself—that you put a lot of time into pleasing you. If he peeps that, he's going to figure automatically that he better get with the program and be ready to please you, too.

So put on that fly suit, the one that hugs your butt just right, shows off those thick legs.

Pick up that curling iron or grab that Kemi oil and tighten up that hair.

Slide a little color on those lips of yours, and hook up those eyes with some mascara.

Square off those shoulders and walk down that street like you own the joint.

Be a fly girl.

True, looks are superficial, and yes, a person should be recognized for the beauty they possess inside rather than out—yadda, yadda, yadda. But the fact remains that physical attraction will be the quickest asset to get you in the brother's door. He's looking for the woman who, like Ralph Wiley wished for in his essay "Dear Jesus," will "make you say 'Damn!,' even if you're in church or with your mother." He wants the woman who is so fine, so well oiled, so completely tuned that she'll have all the brothers whispering their desires for her over the watercooler—even though he doesn't want the fellas talking that kind of talk within his earshot.

And a Sistahs' Rules girl is going to give him just that.

But remember: You're not doing this just for him. Above all else, you're doing this for you. Debrena Jackson Gandy, author of *Sacred Pampering Principles: An African-American Woman's Guide to Self-Care and Inner Renewal,* says that it is of the utmost importance that we sistahs treat ourselves special— get our hair done, dress nicely, pamper ourselves with massages and manicures, and take time to put our spirituality in gear— because once we do, we feel so much better about ourselves.

I know a sistah who doesn't take care to comb her hair as well as she should, who hardly ever dresses up—and even when she does, it's haphazard at best. She mopes around all day, beats herself up for not being as pretty as some of our other friends, and criticizes all our girlfriends for "having it totally together."

And then she laments that she doesn't have a man.

It's not hard to imagine why.

Low self-esteem and self-pity are about as much fun as an early-morning rendezvous with a dentist and a needle full of novocaine. Nobody wants to be around a miserable, busted woman—whether they be a woman or a man. We need to take Debrena's advice: Pamper ourselves, feel better about ourselves. When we get that self-esteem intact, we'll step lively—like we're God's special gift to the world.

The bonus prize here is that black men will pick up on that

vibe and be drawn to it like bees to honey. They'll notice you, compliment you—break their necks to talk to you.

So hook it up, girl.

Spend that extra forty dollars and let the hairdresser wash and set your hair or tighten up those locks. Take the ten dollars you would have spent on a fattening lunch and get your nails done, and spend an extra ten to let the pedicurist work on those toes. Buy that expensive perfumed lotion and slather it all over your body to soften up your skin, make it smell pretty and glow. Join the gym, work out, and firm up that body. Go on down to the Body Shop and buy some of that fragrant raspberry bubble bath and some scented candles, and lose yourself in a luxurious, sensuous bath—alone. Forget the world exists and treat yourself to a weekend at the spa—with no phone, no television, no newspapers.

Get to know yourself—every inch of you.

And above all else, pray for strength and inner renewal. Ask God to come in and help you clean house.

Then stroll into a room crowded with brothers and watch them shower you with the digits.

It's that simple.

There are feminists who will argue that this rule is foolish—that this male-dominated society has hoodwinked us into thinking that if we don't kill ourselves to be beautiful all the time, we won't be accepted by men. Don't wear makeup, they'll scream. Don't be sexy—you don't need to look cute for any man, they'll charge. They'll point you out as a victim—a victim who foolishly lets a man define her beauty.

I say they're more than likely the ones who don't have men, either.

Look, I'm not saying that you have to let beauty define you. Everybody knows that a pretty face doesn't mean a thing when it comes down to the meat of it. Look at Halle Berry; poor girl was all up on *Oprah,* crying and carrying on over her estranged pro baseball player husband, David Justice, and the breakup of their marriage. She's so divinely beautiful, so incredibly perfect that she makes you want to smack her. But there she was, heartbroken, claiming her man made her feel so worthless and lowdown that she was but a fingersnap from committing suicide.

If Halle Berry—arguably the most beautiful woman in the world—could get dissed, then you know there's no guarantee that your man won't dog you. But that's no excuse to look busted. And there's certainly nothing wrong with letting men notice you being cute, dressing nice, and looking good.

Nobody's saying you have to look dip all the time, either.

We're all guilty of backsliding every once in a while. You know, you're making a quick run to the store so you pull your baseball cap over your eyes and double-step it to the corner—praying all the way that your cutie-pie next-door neighbor doesn't come bounding out of his apartment. Or it's dress-down day at work, and you take full advantage of it with some jeans and that easy-to-obtain ponytail 'do.

What's going to separate you from Ms. Ragglely, though, is that your next-door neighbor will already have had a look at you when you were Ms. Fly Girl—so he won't be taken aback by your down days. In fact, he'll probably be turned on by your jeans and sneakers, knowing what you're capable of looking like in that slinky dress and high heels.

So you work it, girl—then sit back and watch them come running.

Get That Wish List in Order

Wanted: A thirty-something single college-educated black male with a six-figure career, a home and luxury car, who is attractive, muscular, family-oriented, trustworthy, honest, church-going, and good in bed.

Just as I was about to write a story about black women and dating for my newspaper, the *Daily News,* I sat a group of my single-and-looking girlfriends down and asked them to come up with a "Wanted" list of characteristics they looked for in their potential Brother Mr. Rights, and this is the consensus they came to. It made for a great lead to my story; so excited was I that I showed it to my editor-in-chief, Pete Hamill.

He read it and burst out laughing.

"Damn. I'd marry him too!"

Indeed, brother would be a perfect catch. He'd just have it all—the house, the car, the titles, the money, the looks—and some morals to boot. Who wouldn't rush him down the aisle?

He's perfect.

Too damn perfect, if you ask me. I mean, are you searching for a good black man or God?

News flash: The last perfect man to walk this earth got nailed to a cross—and he's a little too busy to stroll down the aisle right now.

Don't get me wrong. I know there's a host of black men who fit that wish-list profile, but there's a whole lot of them who don't. Does that mean they're not good men?

Of course not. But we've been brainwashed into thinking that it does.

See, we've gotten used to holding black men to the same rigorous standards that our white counterparts hold their men to—and in the process, we've turned dating into an unrealistic strategic search. Then we get mad when we can't find one who fits the criteria, and go proclaim to the world that there are no good black men.

Hello. Get real.

"This culture has us focused on the bullet point: What does he do, is he financially secure, is he attractive?" Debrena Jackson Gandy told me when I was writing the story for the *News*.

"Those things matter, too, but as people of color, we've always had a spiritual fusion in everything we do, and we have to do that with relationships."

Julia Boyd, a practicing Seattle-based psychotherapist and book author, put it even more bluntly: "I don't want to discourage sisters from having a shopping list. But are you going for name brands only, or do sales attract you too? Because sometimes, sale things aren't a bad deal."

Preach on, sis.

Say he didn't have a college degree and a six-figure salary, that he was a blue-collar worker who drove a Honda instead of a Lexus, but he was attractive, family-oriented, and trustworthy. Would that make him any worse a man than, say, Mr. Super Brother? Say he did have the Lexus and the impressive titles and salary, but he wasn't trustworthy and honest and good in bed. Would he still fit your Super Brother fantasy? Would you be willing to be alone for the rest of your life because the last man you dealt with had all the characteristics you were looking for, except that he wasn't all that attractive?

I would hope not.

See, sometimes you've got to rearrange those priorities, recognize when some things just aren't as important as others—because the fact of the matter is, there are brothers out there who fit that wish list; there just aren't nearly enough to go around.

A Sistahs' Rules girl knows that it's important to prioritize.

Prioritize, prioritize, *prioritize.*

Her wish list is filled with interchangeable preferences; she's willing to make sacrifices for the good of the team. She's willing to wait for the more important characteristics a man has to offer—honesty, trustworthiness, sincerity—and willing to put the more material things—the white picket fence, the garage, and the pool—on the back burner if she recognizes that what she has in front of her is truly a good black man.

I have a girlfriend who isn't willing to heed this advice. She's a great woman, and would make any man happy; she's pretty, sweet, intelligent, hardworking—got a job, with benefits.

And she's always asking folks to hook her up—but she insists that the candidate fit exacting criteria similar to those laid out in the sample wish list at the beginning of this chapter.

She once asked me if I knew any good men I could introduce her to, and one gentleman immediately came to mind, a conductor who collects tickets on the train I ride to work in the morning. On the face of it, he fit a few of her top priorities: He was handsome, muscular, seemed nice, easy to talk to, and he didn't have a ring on his finger—so I assumed he was single. She was open until I mentioned he worked for New Jersey Transit.

"Oh, hell, no. I need a doctor or a lawyer."

I kept insisting that he seemed like a great guy—and deserved a chance.

No dice.

It never occurred to her that the bargain brother may have

made her even more satisfied than the top-shelf super Negro she'd been searching for all her life. She's still waiting for the M.D. and the counselor, moaning about how there're no good black men out there.

I have another friend who won't give a guy so much as a second glance if he has a big stomach. Another friend will immediately head for the other direction if the guy pursuing her doesn't play professional sports. Still another says if he's not dark-skinned, he's not in.

If they're willing to wait it out, that's their prerogative. But their priorities seem a little askew.

Are yours?

Life's a little too short for all that.

I'm not saying that a girl shouldn't have standards; there have to be some boundaries, some lines drawn in the sand. But don't pass on the sale racks; you're probably missing out on some great bargains.

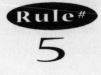

Get Out of His Wallet

If your dream man has Bill Cosby money, then you need to wake up. Camille Cosby, after all, has that man and his bank account on lockdown—and not too many other available black bachelors have that kind of loot.

Not enough, at least, to go around.

Besides, that's the fairy tale white women's Cinderella dreams are made of. They've been conditioned from birth to hold out for that Prince in Shining Armor—the Ward Cleaver who will have the impressive title to go with the impressive job, and can readily afford to give his wife the big house, the fancy car, the expensive clothes, the gold card, the fat bank account, and the nanny to watch the 2.4 kids playing inside the white picket fence.

Of course, in American society the luck of the draw is in white women's favor. The odds are greater for them that they'll find just that kind of guy—mainly because it's white men who dominate the positions that make them society's top money earners.

That's not to say that there aren't any black men with M.D., Ph.D., M.B.A., president, executive director, owner, or attorney-at-law titles following their names. Today, more than ever, black men are snapping up those impressive positions with amazing ease, taking their place among the upper echelons of America.

But chances are more likely than not that your Brother Mr. Right is going to be a diamond in the middle-class or even lower-class rough than he is a Black Prince in a shiny white Mercedes Benz—and you really don't have the kind of time on your hands to be waiting for the latter. What you need to do is get your nose out of his wallet and stop discounting brothers who can't measure up to Cinderella's materialistic fantasies.

If the brother you're interested in has the money, the house, the car, the cards, and the titles, well then, good for you. But does that automatically mean that he's going to treat you right? Does it guarantee that he's going to be caring and sensitive and trustworthy and down for you at all times?

Hell, no—because money doesn't mean anything in the emotional scheme of things.

A Sistahs' Rules girl knows that money is not synonymous with good black men—that the ones who are sincerely good brothers come just as rich as Grant Hill and just as poor as your daddy, can either own the bank or be cleaning it, running the magazine or running the mailroom, teaching the college class or attending it between shifts at the post office. They can be CEOs or COs, psychiatrists and writers or postal men and funeral parlor directors—rich or living paycheck to paycheck. She doesn't care that he doesn't drive a Mercedes, makes five figures instead of six, and lives in a one-bedroom apartment and not a mansion. What she wants is a good man who will be sweet, caring, sensitive, and trustworthy and who will love her unconditionally; she knows that the material things are incidental here.

There isn't a day that goes by that I don't thank God that my mother thought this way. It was 1963. My mother saw my father outside his aunt's house, washing his brown Oldsmobile. She thought he was cute, so she walked on down to the store, switching all the way so that he would notice her. He saw her and whistled. Her smile, he says, was as bright and sweet as the early morning sun. She stopped, they chatted, he promised her a date. That next Saturday, he took her out—nothing fancy, a movie. And when he drove up in front of her house in his brown Oldsmobile, she decided she didn't want the date to end. They sat in that car and talked and talked and talked some more—for hours, until the sun rose. That he was a worker in a plastics factory never fazed her; he was, and still is, a sweet, handsome, generous man who cared about family and loved being in love. My mom says, "He was always a hustler—always made sure that we had food on the table and shoes on our feet. Oh, he was a good provider. Always put his family first."

Still, there are months when he's trying to figure out where he's going to get the money to pay the two mortgages, the water, heat, light and cable bills, the car notes and the insurance—and he and my mother struggle.

Mommy often jokes to my father now that if she knew he wasn't going to be rich and that she would still be working at age fifty-seven, she would have never married him. He says, "Same here." Then they look at each other and burst into laughter. I don't know what those two would have done without each other these last three decades—and I certainly couldn't imagine growing up without such a powerfully sensitive, loving, caring man in my life.

My father is a good, honorable man—the best there is. It was his qualities I searched for when I was looking for an equally good man for myself. You can best bet that my search never started in any man's wallet.

Besides, any black man with money and a little bit of sense is going to know it when you're trying to juice him for his bank. If he's smart, he'll kick your golddigging butt right to the curb—à la Mike Tyson–Robin Givens. Only the sincerely shallow would stay with a woman who's dating him for his money—and if he does stay with her, well then, he deserves what he gets.

I know a girl named Lila whose goal in life was to marry an NFL player. She put herself in all the right situations, all the right social cliques, so that she could snag one. Last year, she finally met this poor fool I'll call Paul up in Cape Cod—and he fell for her hook, line, and sinker. She readily admits that she doesn't love him, but she's got the boy fooled into thinking she really gives a damn because she's more interested in using their relationship to make a profit. She even conned him into giving her an engagement ring.

My girls and I have given that marriage all of a year.

I would hope he has sense enough to get with that pre-nup—but hey, if he was dumb enough to give her a ring, he's dumb enough to show her all his money. Personally, I feel sorry for the boy—knowing that he and she are going to be rich and lonely.

Now, I know some of you sistahs out there who make that good money and have those impressive titles get offended when someone tells you to "date down." I'm not telling you you need to go down to Crenshaw or Rikers Island and give one of those brothers some love. What I am telling you, though, is that if you're discounting the brother who, while you're walking from the subway, says good morning to you as he's delivering the mail or picking up the garbage from your curbside or teaching your kid's kindergarten class, your pool of eligible black bachelors is going to be a helluva lot smaller than it needs to be. It's really hard to swim in shallow waters.

And while you're sitting home next Saturday evening alone with a bowl of popcorn and the remote, another sistah with vision is going to be romancing the guy to whom you didn't give a second glance.

Hope that popcorn tastes good going down.

Use Your Heart and Not Your Eyes

The prayer for "The Good One" usually opens up something like, "Lawd, I swear I'll never ask you for another single, solitary thing if you send me a man that has Wesley's skin and Tyson's eyes and Grant Hill's smile and Evander Holyfield's body and..."

Then, after about five minutes of nonstop begging for the perfect tall, dark, and handsome Black Prince, we end it with, "Oh, and um, make him sweet, loving, and rich. Amen."

I'll admit it with the rest of you: Wesley is beautiful and Tyson is indeed fine, but a good brother doesn't necessarily have to look like either one of them.

We get hung up on looks, though, don't we? Sistahs will knock down ten perfectly decent-looking guys to get to the hardly-ever-existent-and-certainly-almost-never-available super-handsome one, and then wonder why they can't find and don't have a man—let alone a good one. Get more than two of us in a club full of men, and we'll complain to each other about how there's "no cuties in the house," or how there's all of two cuties in the vicinity and "Why won't they talk to me?"

In the meantime, there's a truckload of brothers over there by the bar, sucking on breath mints, sipping on Heinekens, wondering why none of the ladies are giving them any play.

It's because we don't have our priorities straight on our "Good Man Wish Lists"—that's why. We'll lead it off with superficial characteristics we think our man should have—like a gorgeous face and the body of a god—and, in the process, systematically eliminate the all-right-looking men who, if we gave them half a chance, could be absolutely good to and for us.

How do we get over that? First, reprioritize that list. A Sistahs' Rules girl knows that she needs to use her heart, not her eyes, when deciding whom she's going to give her precious dating time to. She doesn't care that he may be a little overweight, shorter than she may have wanted, lighter than she imagined, and only kinda cute when she squints her eyes a bit and tilts her head to the side. She's not stuttin' it because she will have taken the time to check and see if the brother's beautiful where it counts: On the inside. That means he's loving, honest, trustworthy, sweet, sensitive, caring, and quick to please.

Hell, he can look like Dennis Rodman if he's all that! Truth be told, he'll be all the more handsome to you if he is all those things. Who are you to deny yourself a beautiful man like that just because he's not super-fine?

My girl Cheryl knows. Her wish list for an ideal man ran like this: Fine, tall, muscular, stomach cut, preferably bald, dark skin, doe eyes, cute feet, smart, nice, trustworthy. If he didn't fit her bill to a T, she wasn't interested—period. Age thirty-one and a daughter later, she was still single, complaining about how she just couldn't find her dream man and refusing to settle until she found exactly what she wanted.

Lucky for her, one of our mutual friends had common sense enough to set old girl up on a blind date with a guy from her job—a man who broke almost all of Cheryl's wish-list wants. He was tall but definitely not muscular. Downright scrawny would be a more accurate description. He was about as light-skinned as she, which is pretty light, had a headful of hair, and not all that cute if you thought about it hard enough—almost the opposite of any man Cheryl ever prayed for.

But he showed up to that restaurant with flowers, a sweet smile and a temperament to match, good conversation, and intelligence. Later on, Cheryl found out that he was also trustworthy, honest, and ready, willing, and able to treat her the way she deserved to be treated: special. Old boy turned Cheryl out.

I'm not saying that you have to put on your Nikes and sprint toward the ugliest, most out of-shape brother you see; I mean, you do have to, like, look at him. But at the same time, you shouldn't be so quick to dismiss the average-looking brother, because he just might be prepared to work overtime to make you happy. Ditto for physically challenged brothers, and other black men who have disabilities and non-life-threatening diseases.

So while all the other shallow sistahs are sweatin the Tyson lookalike chasing after the tall, skinny chippy with the weave and fake boobs, why don't you cooly saunter on over to the quiet and kinda cute guy over there by the bar—give him a chance.

Let the chippy sweat her hair out chasing after wannabe.

Use What You Got to Get What You Want

This sistah I used to hang with back in the day once told me that if she knew what city/house/club/bar/social gathering/open field all the "good" black men were hanging at, she'd be "the first in line, for real."

It never dawned on her that she's on that line 24–7.

There is no open field where all the good ones congregate; they're on your job, on the train you take to the job, at the bar after you get off the job, in the bowling league, in your church, in your circle of friends.

Beautiful, decent black men are everywhere.

You just need to use your resources to put yourself in contact with them.

Like, did it ever occur to you that the brother over in the men's section at Macy's, going through the collection of Jerry Garcia ties, could very well be a good man? Or the man you keep bumping into at the local video store, or at the car wash, or walking to his car with the cartful of groceries at Pathmark?

Have you ever asked your friends to set you up on dates—or asked one who has a steady to throw a dinner party with her man so that he could invite along some of his boys to meet you and your girls? You know, come to think of it, Mom's pretty good at that stuff, too. Did you ever think to ask her to check out whether any of her friends have some eligible bachelors for sons?

Ever think that the guy you're sitting next to in church would make a mighty fine husband? Or perhaps the single pastor delivering the sermon? Heck, the one person who knows a host of good black men is the reverend!

Ever been to an NAACP convention, or conventions for black journalists, police officers, lawyers, or corrections officers? How about Sinbad's annual HBO soul concert, or *Essence*'s jazzy jam down in Louisiana, or Martha's Vineyard around the summer holidays—out in Oak Bluffs? I can't stress enough how many eligible black bachelors show up to those joints.

Ever ask the owner of your local black bookstore if she's seen any black men snapping up the latest Cornel West or Walter Mosley book? Ever tried hanging out in the electronics, hardware, or sporting goods stores? Ever go check out the baseball game at the park on a sunny Saturday, or the basketball game at the local gym on Thursday afternoon, or the Sunday touch football game? Tons of black men. Good ones.

I'm not saying that you have to turn this into an all-points-bulletin search—but black men aren't just going to fall out of the sky and right into your lap. You simply have to keep your eyes open, work your resources, and use your access to get in touch with what you want—black men. Whether they're good or not you'll have to determine later. What's important is that you put yourself in the places where they're likely to be, that's all.

Of course, there're just some places where you shouldn't even think about looking for a black man—because you'd just be begging for trouble if you did. To help you determine what's safe, I've devised a list of places where it's okay to look for a guy, and places where it isn't exactly the wisest thing to do. Note: Some of the places on the "Don't Step to Him Here" list may be a tad obvious—but damn if some of you all don't need the help.

You Can Meet a Good Brother at:

- The dance club or happy hour at the happening bar
- The job

- Your friend's dinner party
- The wedding reception
- The annual NAACP banquet, the Essence Awards, and other black-tie affairs
- Jamaica and other vacation spots. (Hey, it worked for Terry McMillan, didn't it? Of course, with this one, you may need to cancel out a few of the rules, like Rule #13: No Swerving on the First Date, and Rule #15, The Way to a Man's Heart Is Through a Great Plate of Greens.)
- The grocery store, dry cleaner and other errand spots
- The book store, record store, video store, and other home-entertainment spots
- The mall
- The gym

Don't Try to Meet a Brother at:

- The family reunion. (He could be a cousin or the boyfriend of a cousin. And although it's been fifteen years since she kicked your butt, perhaps you don't want to test her today.)
- The liquor store or any other place where a man is able to buy liquor and there's no dancing involved
- The welfare office
- The clinic
- The C-Lo spot

- The Immigration and Naturalization Service office
- The basketball courts on a weekday afternoon
- The lingerie store
- The perfume counter—anytime outside of two weeks before or after Mother's Day
- The gay dance club or any other establishment with the Gay Pride flag waving outside

Yes, it would be easier if you could just get a postcard in the mail telling you where to show up to meet all of the eligible black bachelors—but that's just not going to happen. Besides, it just wouldn't be much fun. You can, however, learn how to insert yourself into situations where there will be a few to choose from. Get your girlfriends, your mother, your pastor, your local black organization, and your pedicurist on the case. One of them knows your Brother Mr. Right.

Trust me.

Go Get Him, Girl!

You're in the lunchroom at the job, and just as you're waiting for the counter lady to plop that meat-loaf sandwich on that cardboard tray, you look up and see that God has sent through the double doors a gift you are sure was put on this earth especially for you.

He is tall. He is fine. He is in a suit. He has all his teeth.

You look at the counter lady, who, as she dips her hand into the potato chip bowl, winks at you and smiles. You look at the gift again, and vaguely remember some of your colleagues mentioning that there's a new cutie-pie black guy in the advertising department. It's him, you're sure of it. He strolls out before you have the chance to say anything.

If you're a true Sistahs' Rules girl, you're going to find some excuse to go into his office and investigate. You'll check for the ring and survey the landscape for any telltale signs of a mate. If it's all clear, you'll step to him.

That's right—introduce yourself and strike up a conversation.

Why not?

You've got absolutely nothing to lose and everything on this earth to gain. This could well be a potential Brother Mr. Right— and you want first dibs. First dibs never go to the shy girl who sits back and waits to be approached; that act-aloof-and-hope-he-notices-you thing is played like an eight-track. It's just not cute in the nineties, because men can't read that. You might flash him a little back, and look at him and shyly turn your head in the other direction—but today, that's no indication for him that he can talk to you. Indeed, many a brother has been dissed outright for telling a woman she looks nice, or just plain saying hello to a sistah. They're certainly not looking for the opportunity to get dissed, so they may avoid talking to you altogether.

They do like being flattered, though, particularly by a sistah who has confidence enough to smile, say hello, and open up the opportunity—if they're interested—for dating possibilities. It takes the pressure off them; the moment you open your mouth, they'll know you're approachable, that you're not going to dis them the moment they work their mouth to say hello.

It also gets you noticed more quickly—particularly in a club setting, where guys are surrounded by a roomful of women who also might be looking for the opportunity to attract their attention.

Think about it: If you're in a club or in a store or restaurant and you see a guy who floats your boat, the odds are that you will only have one, maybe two shots to connect with each other. You can't pull out a Bible in the club and pray to the Lord that he miraculously walks up to you. And if he doesn't see you, but you notice him and don't speak, that moment of indecision means your potential Brother Mr. Right might just walk out the door without your having given yourself the opportunity to meet him and greet him and check him out.

What's the worst thing that could happen, anyway? Brother could say a cheery "Hello" and introduce you to his date, or you could have missed that gold band on the left ring finger, or he could just make it really clear that he's not interested. Yes, to get your feelings hurt in that situation would kinda suck, but the benefits would far outweigh the negatives—particularly if he bites.

At the very least, you could always have another drink and move on to the next one.

Be careful, though, not to overdo it. They're still men and they still need to feel they've played some part in initiating your groove on. So when you approach him, say "Hello," strike up a conversation, perhaps ask him to dance—but don't ask him out on a date. If he's interested and not a complete numbskull, he'll bite and ask you out on a date—or at least offer up the digits.

If he asks for your number, give him the digits to the office, and plan for a lunch date—so that you can check him out in the light. You don't want any booger bears showing up on your doorstep.

But you do eventually want to get someone there—so you take the initiative and introduce yourself. I assure you, you'll never have another lonely night if you master the art.

My girl Tee could give lessons on this. I mean, homegirl is so good that all of my girlfriends swear up and down they want to be just like her when they grow up. Really, she's good—I've seen her in action. We were out on Thanksgiving night, full from turkey and stuffing and collard greens, getting our groove on at this exclusive Philadelphia nightclub, when Tee spotted out this handsome man across the room. We knew she was interested in him just by the gleam in her eye; he'd set off her cutie-pie alarm in a big way. Of course, there were about a billion other women in the joint who knew who he was, too, but none of them—and certainly none of us—had the cojones to let him catch us looking anywhere within a five-mile radius of where he was standing, let alone make eye contact with him.

Not my girl Tee, though. Girlfriend surveyed the room, smoothed down her little dress, puffed up her hair, and put on her prettiest dimpled smile—and walked right on over to where the boy was standing, near the bar. She didn't say anything at first, just asked the bartender for a white wine. While she was waiting for her drink, she casually and nonchalantly turned to her left and smiled at him. Ol' boy smiled right back. She turned back quickly, searching for the bartender with her wine. Then, slowly, she looked at him again. He smiled again and took the last swig of his beer. "Looks like you're all out," she said, pointing at his empty mug. "May I buy you another?" Ol' boy was flabbergasted; not only was she fine, but she was offering to buy *him* a drink. Just for G. P. he was going to talk to her, because it never happened like this for him. Women walked up to him and asked him to buy them a drink all the time, then walked away like they'd just pumped two quarters in the soda machine and got their Coke and were in need of nothing else. But this one, she was pretty, she had a killer smile, and she was flipping the script on him with the "Can I buy you a drink?" line. She reached into her purse to pay for the drink, but being the gentleman that he was, he told her the beer and wine were on him. She thanked him, and introduced herself. They exchanged a few pleasantries between sips of their drinks, then headed straight for the dance floor.

Here it is almost six months later, and she's making plans to go see him down in Texas, where, it turns out, ol' boy plays for a professional football team during the NFL season. On his off time, he's in Philly, chillin' with my girl Tee.

It's that simple.

And to think girlfriend didn't even have to put up the four-fifty for that Heineken!

If He Gives You a Pager Number Instead of the Digits, Dump His Butt

(And Other Recognizable Signals That Indicate You Need to Kick Him to the Curb)

In every aspect of life, there are going to be winners and there are going to be losers.

Black men are no exception.

Certainly, there is a cadre of brothers out there who are ready, willing, and able to make us happy, those who take care of themselves and their families, are attentive to our needs, respect us as sistahs and lovers, and do everything within their power to be the strong black men we need them to be.

But, Lord, if there aren't some doozies out there who haven't a clue! You know the kind: The inconsiderate / no-job-having / uneducable / immature / out-of-shape / can't-dress / mentally unstable / disrespectful / drug-addicted / no-manners-and-no-clue-about-romance / kid-hating / disheveled-stinky-and-proud-of-it / playa-from-the-Himalaya who always wants to roll up in your direction and block your view while you're in the process of looking for a good brother.

A few of us see him when he's strolling in our direction—and we either run like hell or we handle it accordingly, then move on to the next one. But some of us haven't a clue when the foul winds of planet Bad Brother are about to blow him right in our direction.

Admittedly, there's some gray area in determining whether he's good enough for you; a true Sistahs' Rules girl knows that she has a wish list to stick to, and that there's no universality in the characteristics that make one brother good enough for one woman and not the next.

Some things, though, you just have to say no to—refuse to tolerate. So, written especially with you sistahs in mind—a tip sheet for recognizing he's no damn good.

You know you need to dump his butt if:

- You turn out the lights and something in his mouth sparkles. (I mean, there's plenty of benefit to being able to see your man in the dark—but damn, you gotta bring him home to Mom.)

- He's still rocking that greazy ass jherri curl (the pillow cases, y'all—the pillow cases).
- His hair is long and thick enough for a pick, but he apparently doesn't use one.
- If the words "yo" and "baby" appear anywhere in the first two sentences he says upon his initial attempt to secure the digits.
- He tells you, upon first meeting you, "You kinda cute—for a dark-skinded girl."
- He looks at your natural or your dreads and offers you the number of a beautician who does "great relaxers"—without your having asked for the info.
- He appears to have all the couth—or the lack thereof—of Jerome in the television show *Martin* ("I said Jerome in da howse!")
- His idol was Superfly and he pays daily tributes to him by wearing a butterfly collar, a floor-length coat, and one of those big-ass fedoras. (Ron O'Neil and Sinbad are the only exceptions to this rule.)
- The all-important sneaker-to-shoe ratio exceeds one pair of sneakers to every two pair of shoes. (The only possible exception is a pro ball player, and even then, maybe not.)
- His wardrobe seems to consist exclusively of outfits that lack a belt and feature at least four inches of his boxers showing above his precariously drooping pants.
- A good 50 percent of the hangers in his closet are occupied by a wide assortment of sweatshirts with hoods.

- You find yourself holding your breath when you walk into his apartment and leave hoping like hell you don't smell like that when you get outside.

- Before he agrees to take a trip with you, he says he needs to ask his mama.

- He goes to sleep in a fetal position, curled around the basketball.

- You beep him and a woman calls you back and says, "Who the hell are you and why are you beeping my man?"

- He has a tan line on his left ring finger.

- He tells you he would have graduated from high school but he left in protest because the teachers were racist.

- His idea of following current events is checking today's lottery numbers.

- You open up the cabinet and he has his own collection of paper bags to hold his 40s.

- When you drive by the liquor store, he does the sign of the cross.

- You spot him standing on the corner more than twice on your way home from work (big indication that he has an assigned "Just Chillin'" post there).

- He calls your house at three A.M. on a Tuesday, talking about he's chillin' with the fellas.

- You call the number he marked "work" on that little piece of paper he gave you at the club, and nobody in the office has ever heard his name.

- Whenever a cop car drives by, he slouches in his seat and pulls his hat down over his face.
- The first time you two argue, the word "bitch" shows up anywhere in the conversation.
- You notice that when he gets upset, his fist manages to connect with the wall.
- You notice that his therapist is on speed-dial.
- He brings groceries to your house and puts his name on the orange juice.
- He tries to set up a date so you can buy furniture for his apartment.
- He elbows you from in front of the mirror more than once.
- The last time he saw a sit-up was when he was reaching for the remote at the foot of the bed.
- He pulls up to your house pumping Garth Brooks on his stereo.
- For him, adequate foreplay is unzipping his pants and turning off the lights.
- The amount of time it took for you two to have sex makes you want to run over to the clock and check to see if the big hand still works.
- When the subject of oral sex comes up, he says, "Eew, no way in the world I'd put my face down there!"
- He tells you, "It just doesn't feel as good with it on."

If He Sends You Flowers Just Because, He Could Be a Keeper

(And Other Recognizable Signals That Indicate He's Your Potential Brother Mr. Right)

He's not hard to recognize.

In fact, if you know what you're looking for—and you don't let those superficial desires cloud your judgment—you'll find that a good brother is easier to spot than you've ever imagined. All it takes is an open mind, an ounce of faith, and a little nudge in the right direction by yours truly.

The key here is to remember that the yardstick by which you measure him does not include money, societal status, or potential for your own personal material gain; only Barbie checks for that. What we're looking for is a different kind of breed—the considerate/hardworking/reasonably educated/mature/sexy/mentally stable/respectful/clean/drug- and prison-record-free/fun/honest/ trustworthy brother who will make us, as Terry McMillan so aptly put it, "exhale." That means he may not be all that cute, he may not drive a Mercedes, and he may not be able to take you to the fanciest restaurants, but damn if he doesn't make you feel like you're the queen of Egypt.

That's right—they're out there, sistahs. So get your pen out and check off the tips that apply to your man.

You'll know he's a potential Brother Mr. Right if:

- He loves God, and recognizes that there is a higher being in control of our destinies.
- He has neat hair, nails, toes, and clothes and is concerned— but not overly concerned—about looking good.
- The first time he speaks to you, he does so with the utmost respect. ("Good morning, sistah, how are you today?" is a pretty good one.)
- When he steps to you in the club, he introduces himself and offers to buy you a glass of wine.
- When he asks you to dance, he doesn't rub all over your body on the dance floor, and after you're finished, he thanks you for your company.
- He's just as comfortable with your natural and dreads as he is with your relaxer or weave.

- He wears Armani, but looks just as good in one of those JCPenny specials.
- He's just as comfortable in shoes as he is in sneakers.
- He not only knows how to tie a tie, but actually likes wearing them.
- He hasn't lived with his mama in years.
- He's independent, but still helps his mom out from time to time.
- His apartment is a bachelor's pad—but it's clean, smells decent, and there's at least one place for you to sit besides the bed.
- His medicine cabinet has dental floss, toothpaste, cologne, and other toiletries.
- He lets you answer his phone and his door, and he gives you access to his E-mail account. (No man with something to hide would allow that!)
- He gives you a key to the crib and the car.
- He lets you drive the car.
- He lets you spend the night and doesn't push you to do anything.
- He draws you a hot bath after a hard day's work and goes out of his way to pamper you when you've had a really bad one.
- He makes breakfast with you in the morning, or he makes it for you altogether.
- He's spontaneous.
- He gives you the numbers to his home, work, and pager—and they all work.
- He tells you up front that he's dating other women.

- He drops them all because he really likes you more.
- He's up on current events—and can discuss them with ease.
- He can argue the merits of using Ebonics in the classroom—in the King's English.
- He drinks his beer from bottles no bigger than twelve ounces.
- The only white powder he's ever come in contact with is flour and sugar.
- His cigars are filled with nothing more than tobacco.
- The only time you see him on the corner is when he's buying milk from the local bodega.
- He never calls you or any other woman a bitch or ho.
- He never uses his hands or fists to express his anger.
- When he argues with you—he is able to end it by being able to agree to disagree, and moving on.
- He's trustworthy.
- He's honest with you—but knows the perfect way to do it without being insulting.
- He works out regularly, but doesn't take it to extremes.
- He has friends and spends quality time with them—but not so much that he forgets about you.
- Your mother likes him.
- His musical tastes are diverse.
- You feel like you can learn from him, and he's not afraid to learn a few things from you.
- He's sexy as hell and makes you want to break down and be a freak mama.

- He's just as intent on pleasing you with foreplay as he is with achieving orgasm.
- He likes oral sex—and loves performing it.
- He always wears a condom, and has them readily available.
- He's into round one, round two, and round three—and really has no problem doing it all night long.
- He appreciates the special things you do for him—and never takes them for granted.
- He sincerely gets along with most of your girlfriends.
- He sends flowers to the job—just because.
- He makes you laugh.
- He loves kids.
- He's a good father to his own kids.
- He has a respect for our culture, and dedicates some of his time to its uplift.
- He's a role model for young brothers looking for someone to show them how to be men.
- He makes an honest living and isn't ashamed of his profession—even if others are.
- He's not bothered by sharing household responsibilities.
- If he doesn't know how to fix it, he will readily hire someone who can—and not be embarrassed by it.
- If he's lost, he'll pull over and ask for directions.
- He tells you you're beautiful—even on your ugly days.

Call the Brother, Date the Brother

To hell with holding on to his number and waiting for him to call you three times before you return his phone call. Ditto for accepting Saturday dates only before Wednesday and restricting yourself to seeing him only once a week.

What on earth is the point?

Brothers don't want to have to be put through all those rigid, ridiculous paces to speak to or see a sistah. Remember: they're just as insecure and unsure about new relationships as we are; the dating game is fraught with just as many neuroses and insecurities for them as it is for us. So they take every bit of information, every move you make, as a sign of whether or not they're about to get a chance with you or get dissed. If you're not returning his phone calls and you're making it hard for him to see you, what kind of message are you sending to him?

The kind that alerts his "I'm About to Be Dissed" sensor, no doubt.

Chances are, he's going to figure you don't want to be bothered—because that's the kind of behavior you save for someone you don't want to be bothered with. If you didn't want to be bothered with him, you shouldn't have given up the digits in the first place—or you should at least give him the courtesy of returning his phone call and telling him that now is just not the right time for you to start any new relationships.

Anything less than that is just plain rude.

Besides, there's nothing a black man hates more than a sistah who plays games. He's not dumb; he figures out those artificial time lines you've established to reel him in and quickly determines that they are superficial and fake at best, and at worst, a ploy by you to rope him into a relationship he may not be ready for. He's figuring, "Damn, I just wanted to take the sister out, show her a good time, perhaps have some good conversation—that's all." He figures if he has to toss himself through all those hoops to get you just to go out on a date with him, or engage in a simple phone conversation, what on earth will he have to put himself through in a full-time relationship with your game-playing behind?

He'll quickly determine it's just not worth the effort—particularly if there's another woman who is giving him a little play, and who takes special care not to be so rude as to not return a phone call or consistently turn down dates just to be turning them down.

Look at it like this: You get your hair done, you put on makeup, and you slide into one of your sexiest outfits and go out to the club with your girls. You all line up next to the dance floor and proceed to talk about people and scowl at any man who deigns even to work his mouth to look like he's about to ask one of you to dance. He recognizes it, and moves on to the sistah standing next to you all—the one who's smiling, enjoying the music, and dancing in place. She's approachable, and he approaches. They hit the floor and have a good old time, while you and your girls complain about how nobody's asked you all to dance.

Can you blame him for moving on to the next one? Well, the same thing applies to a sistah who doesn't return phone calls and makes it overly difficult for him to see her. Sure, the guys like the chase, but how hard must a guy run to get the sistah he likes to use her dialing finger or go out on a date with him? After a while, he'll simply pack up his gym shoes, and take his game somewhere else. Brothers just don't need to—and won't—put themselves through all that artificial dog training.

That's not to say that you should make it all easy for the brother. If he calls you after your lunch break on Friday and says he wants to take you out Friday night, go with him if you really want to go that night. But don't let him make that a habit. In fact, you should allow it only once—and only if you have absolutely nothing else planned. And you should never, under any circumstances, cancel plans that you've made with others to go out with a man. Unless, that is, he's given you a decent amount of notice that he wants to take you out and you really want to go out with him rather than sit at your friend's house playing bid whist with the girls.

But if he calls you after Wednesday and before Friday lunch break and says he's got, say, two tickets to a concert and invites you to come with him, and you have nothing else to do and no other plans, go. It beats the hell out of sitting home on a Friday night by yourself. Plus, you don't want him taking some other babe to the concert—which you know he'll do because he's not going to let his ticket go to waste. Wouldn't it make more sense if you're the sistah he takes to the concert—if you're the one spending the evening charming his socks off and having a good time? You have much more control over whether he takes you out again if you work it right on those first few dates than you have sitting home watching HBO and eating popcorn while he's out with some other woman who was smart enough to take advantage of the situation and go.

I guarantee you that when he's out with her, he won't be thinking about you—the rude sistah who can't return phone calls and keeps rejecting his offers for a good time.

HOW TO GET A GOOD BLACK MAN

How to Work It on Your First Few Dates, Before You Get to Doing the Nasty

So you sealed a date. You go, girl!

Now you just have to know how to work it.

The key here is to put this dating thing in proper perspective: The first few meetings between you two are the discovery/exploration phase—the time in which you'll learn about each other's common interests, goals, and aspirations, backgrounds and worldviews. It's when you find out if you two click. You want to use this opportunity to determine if you can get along with this person well enough to consider a long-term relationship with him, or if he's a fool who needs to be fired, quick, fast, and in a hurry. He's going to use this as his opportunity to determine if he likes you and wants to see you again, or if he's just going to try to hit it on occasion and save the good stuff—his commitment—for someone else.

Neither of you will know which category the other will fall in until the first few dates are behind you. Simply put: The first three dates are crucial. You've got to know how to act, and recognize the signs.

Let him pick where you two will dine, and insist that you meet him there. This way, when the date is over, you can go your way and he can go his—and neither of you will be tempted to come to the other's house for a nightcap. (We want to avoid any temptations to break Rule #13: No Swerving.)

On your first date, show up looking sexy as hell and acting as down-to-earth as if you've been his homie for years. This is a date, not a job interview; you're there to have fun. Keep the serious stuff to a minimum, and focus on the fun things you have in common. Laugh at his jokes and make some of your own. Talk about your jobs, where you grew up and the neighborhoods you live in—but avoid telling him about your screwy co-worker, your brother's prison record, or how much your sister fights with her husband. Discuss current events, but avoid topics that would lead you into a debate over ideology. You don't give a damn that he's a Republican just yet. He doesn't care that you showed up to the junior high at 6:00 A.M. to pull the voting lever for Clinton. This is a getting-to-know-the-cool-side-of-you date, not a historic meeting to solve the Middle East crisis. Talk about art, talk about your love for cooking, talk about Spike Lee—and see if he rolls with you in the conversation. Be yourself—because you don't want to be uncomfortable trying to be somebody that you're not, and he doesn't want to be tricked into thinking you're one kind of person, when you're really another.

Above all else, just have a good time—without wondering if he's "The One," how he would propose, or what your children would look like. You're making a new friend—and that's it. Remember that you can't possibly know after three hours what kind of man a complete stranger is. That takes time.

Special note: Show up to the date ready, willing, and able to pay for your meal and entertainment. My mother always told me, when I was going on a date, to keep some money in my wallet in case he was so incredibly simple that I had to leave his butt where he was sitting and find my own way home. "You don't want to have to depend on him for anything," she would always tell me. Today, however, having money in your pocket and the ability and willingness to pay your way shows a brother you're not trying to juice him for his bank—that you're not overly concerned with what's in his wallet. Black men like that, because it shows that you're an independent sistah who isn't depending on a brother to finance her nightly rendezvous.

If he's a good man, he'll probably pay anyway—and you, by all means, should let him. Hey, you're no fool. But as he plunks down the loot for that shrimp scampi dinner you just ate, feel comfortable in the fact that he's just delivered to himself a mental note that you were kind enough to offer to pay your own way. There's nothing wrong with getting on his good side early.

By the end of that date, it's going to be pretty obvious to both of you whether or not you want to do it again. If you were engaging and witty and sexy and down-to-earth, chances are you're probably in there. You'll know he has a remote interest in you if he asks you out again. If you like him, see him—but don't take that as a sign that he's going to ask for your hand in marriage. Recognize it for the signal that it is: He wants to see you again. That's it. Go about the business of dating other men until you come to the mutual conclusion that you are right for each other.

Also, don't be afraid to ask and take him out, either. Brothers dig sistahs who are decisive and can take control of a situation—without being controlling. It's also a good way to find out if he's interested; if he keeps coming up with excuses for why he can't go out, then catch the next bus out of that relationship and roll on to the next.

Use the next few dates to get to know him a bit better, and to reveal a little bit more about yourself. Take the exploration to another level and see if you two can hang. I'm not saying you have to find out what he'd name his firstborn son, but you want to know some basic stuff about him: Is he churchgoing or an atheist? Does he think Newt Gingrich is a god, or does he think voting is a crock? These are things that are going to help you and him determine if the two of you can deal with each other on levels other than superficial—or if this is going to be strictly physical.

You're obviously shooting for the former, so choose wisely.

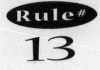
No Swerving on the First Date

He took you out and bought you a nice dinner, you sipped cognac by candlelight, stared deeply into each other's eyes, and held hands in the car all the way home.

He gets out of his ride, opens your door for you, and walks you to your apartment.

He touches your face tenderly, and you lay a kiss on him that has all the heat and passion of one of Marvin Gaye's racier tunes. You pull yourselves away from each other and giggle.

He asks if he can come up for a nightcap—"Just a nightcap, really."

What do you do?

Need you ask? There's only one answer: Tell

him—in a nice way if you think you like him and want to see him again—to get to steppin'. You are to have no nookie on the first date. Ever. No matter how much your hot butt wants to.

Sistahs' Rules girls know they just can't go out like that if they want him to come back—and particularly if they want him to keep them in the running for a serious relationship. Although they wouldn't object outright to boning you on the first date, brothers will always remember in the back of their minds that you are not to be given serious consideration as "The One" later on down the line because you made it really easy for him to have sex with you. Your rendezvous, no matter how spectacular it may be, will be a constant reminder to him that you probably have slept with other men on the first date, too.

This is not a good thing.

What you want is for him to look forward to seeing you again—to think about what your next date will be like, to ponder in his mind what he'll have to do to get some. You want to be—and you want him to believe you to be—a nice girl who has enough sense to know that sex shouldn't come that easy for anybody, no matter how good a brother he might appear to be.

More important here is that you feel comfortable sleeping with him. You want to know in your heart that what you did with him wasn't a mistake—that you have no regrets. You will never, ever feel that way if you give it up right out the box.

Above all else, never make the tragic mistake of equating sex with love. You're a big girl and you should know by now that sex is sex—and for a black man, emotions are hardly ever tied to his penis. For him, sex is purely physical. Just because you're good at it won't mean he'll commit, unless it's absolutely incredible—the best he's ever had and the best he thinks he'll ever have. Of course, skills that fabulous are rare, unless you make a career out of starring in films with names like *Debbie Does Dallas* or *Chocolate Cheerleaders*. So unless your name is Vanessa Del Rio, you'll do well to remember sex means almost nothing in the big picture.

The first time you have sex with him, you should be doing it because you want to take your intimacy to another level—not because you think he loves you and you love him. You want to do more than kiss and hug, but less than have his baby and get married. Nothing more, nothing less. The moment you start tying in all that other emotional baggage is the moment you're going to get your feelings hurt.

We're trying to avoid that at all costs.

I'd suggest you keep it on lockdown at least through the third date—which should give you enough time to figure out if it's something you really, really want to do, and him enough time to feel comfortable that you didn't just fall right into his bed. But never hold out just because you think it's cool to make him wait. Remember: Your holding out isn't going to make him want you more; he can get it elsewhere. The ideal scenario here is if you want to do it with him and he wants to do it with you—and neither of you is expecting anything from the other but a good time. Let all that other stuff—the emotions, the ring, the "I do's"—come later. Much later.

If, after all the preaching I've done, you still won't sleep with a man unless you love him, then you don't need to be sleeping with a man unless you are absolutely, positively, 100 percent without a shadow of a doubt sure that he loves you back—period. That means he put a ring on your finger and you all have taken the blood test and are about to walk down the aisle.

This is a beautiful thing, indeed—but I took a survey and my girls think the last time that's happened was sometime in the early fifties.

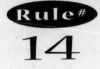
Blow His Mind

There's nothing on this earth that can rival romance—that tingling you get in your stomach when a man unexpectedly sends a beautiful bouquet of roses to your office, or surprises you with a picnic in the park after Sunday service.

It makes you feel special—like a proud peacock turned on by the beautifully colored feathers of its mate. You look forward to the time you spend with him, because you want to feel that way again, and again, and again. You smell the sweet flowers, or gaze into his eyes and start figuring he's got to be jelly, 'cause jam don't make your heart shake like this.

And then, like an insensitive boob, you ruin it

by dismissing the fact that he has feelings, too, and you don't return the favor.

There's a reason for it. Society dupes us, from when we are wee-bit little girls, into thinking that Ken is supposed to pick up Barbie in the fly sports car, flowers in hand, and whisk her away to an exclusive restaurant where he will spend nearly every dime he has in his pocket on her—and all Barbie has to do is sit back, be pleased, and if she feels like it, throw in a thank you and a polite peck on the cheek. Her credo: "You don't owe him anything."

True, you don't owe any man anything. But Sistahs' Rules girls know that successful relationships are grounded on basic give-and-take—the please and be pleased rule. You can't think for a second with black men that you have the "We Need to Be Romanced" department on lockdown. Brothers want, and need, to be romanced, too—no matter how hard or unfeeling they, and society, try to make them out to be. They like the smell of flowers, but enjoy even more the woman who sweeps aside all those ignorant notions that suggest men shouldn't be made to feel special every once in a while. To them, that woman is, indeed, a rare bird.

So be that rare bird for a change. On your first date, bring him flowers—then sit back and marvel in the glow of the smile you put on his face. For every three times he does something romantic for you, return the favor and do at least one thing romantic for him. If he's not very romantic, then you set the example for him by being romantic. In no time, you will get into the habit of pleasing one another—and your potential Brother Mr. Right will know he has a sweet, thoughtful, special woman on his hands.

Of course, there are potential hazards here. You could run into a no-good son-of-a-you-know-what who could mistake your kindness for gullibility—and try to take advantage of it. A leech is a good thing to waste, and you should know how to handle that fool accordingly (see Sistahs' Rule #37). But don't let that stop you from treating the next potential Brother Man right.

Neither he, nor you, after all, deserves anything less.

A friend of mine, Michael, swears he fell in love with his fiancée, Denise, the day she surprised him with a romantic scavenger hunt on New Year's Eve. Five minutes after Denise supposedly left Michael's apartment to run to the store for some juice, his next-door neighbor rang his bell and handed him a red rose and a card that instructed him to go to the video store for his first "clue." There, Michael picked up an erotic video and a second card that instructed him to go to the liquor store for a bottle of Moët. In about an hour's time, Michael made five different stops, picking up, in addition to the video and champagne, a sexy nightgown, a box of Godiva chocolate-covered cherries, and whipped cream. When he went back to his apartment—upon the instructions of his last "clue"—he found Denise sitting in a candlelit bathroom with a bowl of fresh raspberries in hand and a hot, fragrant bubble bath drawn just for him.

Needless to say, they spent New Year's Eve at home.

He proposed three months later. How could he not? he asked. No woman had ever put more than two seconds' thought into doing anything that sweet for him. He spent all the time, energy, and money romancing womenfolk. Then came Denise, who, along with being romanced, enjoyed romancing him.

Their wedding was beautiful.

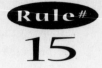

The Way to a Man's Heart Is Through a Great Plate of Greens

Old-fashioned, yes. But trust me—as sure as the sky is blue and Brian McKnight is fine, black men are more apt to fall in love with a woman who can cook them up a nice meal.

The reasons are simple:

• A good home-cooked meal reminds him of home in general, and Mom in particular.

• He's turned on by a woman who will invest time and energy in pleasing him.

• It's yet another thing he can brag about to his mom when he hints he may have found the one.

Now, I know what you independent nineties girls are thinking: Standing over a hot stove for any man other than your daddy or your child went out with Afros and the bump. In the name of shedding that Suzie Homemaker role our moms played during our childhood, we proudly forsake everything that has anything remotely to do with grocery stores, pots, and stoves for take out, TV dinners, and fabulous meals at the local soul food restaurant.

But in our quest to overcome the "barefoot, pregnant, and in the kitchen" role saddled on us by yesteryear's "This Is a Man's World" hierarchy, we lost sight of the fact that the time and effort we put into preparing a good meal for someone special is truly one of the best gifts we could ever give from the heart. Celebrated poet Nikki Giovanni wrote in "The Only True Lovers Are Chefs or Happy Birthday Edna Lewis" that cooking is "love alright cause that other stuff anybody can do and if you do it long enough you can do it either well or adequately but cooking///now that is something you learn from your heart."

Just think about this: How would you feel if you met a man at his house for an early afternoon date, and brotherman surprised you with homemade cinnamon waffles, scrambled eggs, and freshly squeezed orange juice? After you picked your face up off the floor, thanked him, and ate, you'd probably give him some. Admit it: It would be an extremely sweet thing for him to do.

Well, single brothers feel the same way. Chances are that

the swinging bachelor you're interested in has spent so much money in McDonald's that he's a Happy Meal short of owning stock in the joint. He more than likely fiends for home-cooked meals. He knows that love can be found in freshly made creamed corn and fried chicken wings soaked in buttermilk—made by a lover's hand. Nobody has to tell him that the woman who will bend over a sink for an hour or two scraping the grit off those collard greens—who will stand over the stove watching them slow boil over a low fire all afternoon—is a sweet, one-of-a-kind girl, just like his mama.

This, dears, is a good thing. A very good thing. You want to take any good comparisons to Mom that you can get—and this one is the easiest, by far.

Angela knew this much when she was courting Rudy. Girl-friend couldn't boil water without a fourteen-step instruction guide—but she was well aware that one of the many roads to Rudy's heart was paved with plates full of roast beef, well-seasoned greens, and the cheesiest of cheesy macaroni and cheese, his favorite meal. So at least twice a month, she would enlist her friend Anne to come over to her apartment and whip up the meal for her so that she could at least pretend like she knew how to handle herself in the kitchen. While Anne was burning in the kitchen, Angela would be in the back room freshening up her makeup, fixing her hair, and sliding into a sexy outfit. And just before Rudy rang the doorbell, Angela would kick Anne out, then throw a little flour on her chin—à la *I Love Lucy*—to make her intended believe she was the one who'd cooked. When he walked through the door, Rudy would breathe in the aroma of all that good food on the stove, kiss Ms. Angela, sit down to a magnificent dinner, then thank her accordingly.

Of course, that she was kitchen-challenged came out shortly before the wedding—but by then, it didn't matter because he loved her, despite the fact that the only meal she could handle was burned toast and orange juice from concentrate. To him, it was still a meal made with loving hands. His mother, who thought Angela's kitchen strategy was brilliant, now cooks enough on Sundays to feed her, her husband, her son, and her new daughter-in-law—whom she absolutely adores.

Time keeps me from cooking as much as I'd like, but when I do cook for my man, he appreciates it. Every once in a while, I'll cook enough for him to get his fill at the dinner table one night, and pack a lunch for himself for work the next day. He comes home telling me that the guys at the job want to know where they can find a woman who can cook hickory-smoked chili like me—so that they can get down on their knees and put a ring on both her finger and her pots.

Remember this: A Sistahs' Rules girl knows that in a healthy black-on-black relationship, both parties have to be willing to please and be pleased. In doing that, you're going to have to let go of a few of those white feminist notions that suggest "real" women don't care about a man's feelings or his needs or his desires—or his stomach.

Besides, cooking—from the shopping, to the chopping, to the sizzling in the pan—is amazingly relaxing. I love being in a kitchen, just me and my pots, pouring and mixing and stirring and creating with food and seasonings; it's my special quiet time. And when it's time to put that food on the plate and get it on the table and smell the flavors and watch the steam and check out the look on my baby's face when I set this magnificent plate of food before him—it does my heart something lovely. As corny as it may sound, I feel like I'm doing something life-giving—that I've just created something special for us. You and your man just may feel the same way.

So find out what his favorite dish is, get those pots clinking, and invite that man over for some grub. If he's a really good man, he'll return the favor—and you can thank each other accordingly.

Grab a Playbook and Learn Michael Jordan's Moves

Fact: Sistahs can compensate for a whole lot of physical and personality flaws if they let a brother know they like sports. Black men are absolutely fascinated with sistahs who can not only understand the games, but can intelligently discuss basketball, football, baseball, soccer—or anything else, for that matter, that has anything remotely to do with a ball and rough play.

Now, I recognize that for a lot of us, sports aren't exactly high up on the "Things We Most Appreciate" list. But a true Sistahs' Rules girl knows that sports are as necessary to black men as hot sauce and white bread are to fried fish sandwiches.

One simply cannot exist without the other.

Hey, it's in their nature. Society taught us to like dolls, pink, dress-up, and ballet, and to immediately label any girl who likes playing sports a tomboy. Boys were socialized to think that dolls suck, dancing is for sissies, and real guys spend every minute of playtime either competing with or kicking the hell out of their homies.

Now that we're all grown, most of us sistahs still can't stand sports except to check out the cuties. We look up at the television in the bar, see Michael Jordan, comment on how fine he looks in those little red, black, and white shorts, and then two minutes later, we move on to the next subject. If we want to see his Airness again, we peep his picture in a magazine; no need to waste good bar time in front of the television set watching him run up and down the court.

But for brothers, sports are sacred. They spend quality time either playing, watching, or talking about them. They block out two, sometimes three nights a week so that they can run up and down the court or the field or around the baseball diamond with their buddies. If they're going out with the guys to a bar on game night, they know to pick one with a television set—so they won't miss a single play. Before they survey the date landscape, they clutch their Hennessey and their Heineken and they argue over whether Evander Holyfield can indeed kick Mike Tyson's ass a second time and whether any one of the NFL teams will break down and hire a black coach. They lament that Patrick Ewing just might die an eighty-year-old center for the

New York Knicks without having won a championship ring, and they talk incessantly about Michael Jordan's agility—his ability to, tongue wagging, fly through the air and come crashing down on his opponents' necks as he dunks for two more points. They've played these games before, and they know it takes an extraordinary person to be able to do what Ewing and Holyfield and Air Jordan do. They're mesmerized by their skills. They're proud of the fact that those are black men out there on those courts and on those fields, representing black folks. And they use those special moments with the guys to bond, and to stroll down memory lane, remembering what it was like when they were able to play long and hard just like Patrick and Evander and Mike, when they were kids.

Now imagine you, with your sexy self and your white wine, strolling up in between all those cutie-pie, eligible black bachelors and cursing out the ref for not calling a technical when Detroit's Grant Hill was flagrantly fouled on a breakaway, or proudly announcing that Tyson will lose again because he's an inside fighter who isn't used to battling boxers who use their long reaches.

Oh, they'll look at you gapjawed at first. A drink or two might spill.

Perfectly normal.

To the black male sports lover, you will be an enigma—a beautiful freak of nature that indeed is a sight to behold. And one, if not all, will notice you immediately.

I know a sistah, Sherrie, who uses this tactic to break the

ice with brothers. She'll scope out the places where black men are likely to gather, situate herself on the stool or couch or what have you, and keep her eyes trained on the television set. When out of the corner of her eye she sees a cutie walk up, she'll shout out a call to the TV, or comment about a play—and without fail, the brother she's been scoping out will strike up a conversation. Sometimes, she says, he's testing her knowledge of the game, but most of the time he's just shocked that she knows anything about it. The fact still remains that she's struck up a conversation with a man she probably wouldn't have talked to under any other pretense.

For lessons, get a couple of your male buddies, your dad, or your girlfriends who know about sports to teach you what's going on. You don't have to memorize the playbook or anything—but you should understand that there are four quarters to every basketball game, that you have to go ten yards in one down in a football game, and that there are nine innings in baseball. Learn a couple of the players' names, and get to know enough about their skills that you can participate if they come up in conversation. Don't ever, however, paint yourself into a corner, where you make it seem like you know everything about every sport. In fact, you might, after you've revealed to him that you have at least a passing interest, ask him for lessons—or get him to take you to a game or two to learn about it firsthand. Not only will you be participating in something he likes, but you'll get to go out with him and have fun in an environment other than the stale dinner/drinks date.

This rule must, in some shape, form, or fashion, remain in effect even after you get the guy, too. Oh, he'll love you for plenty of other reasons beside your love of sports, but he'll appreciate you even more if, on Super Bowl Sunday, you're contributing more to the game than some hot wings and nachos. He'll brag about you to his friends.

For those of you who just can't stomach the idea of watching the game with the guys, you all must remember that just because you don't like sports doesn't mean you try to stop him from liking sports, too. There's a group of white women who, every Super Bowl Sunday, meet in the city and lament over how their husbands and mates don't pay attention to them when the big game is on. They smash televisions, they nag and complain, and they call the television cameras and newspapers to document it all.

Big mistake. Big. Brothers just don't play that, because they're figuring that if they've spent all week in your face, they should be granted at least one day of peace and quiet with their heroes.

If you're in a committed relationship with a black man, you'll earn major cool points with him if, on the Sunday afternoons when he's glued to the remote and clicking continuously between the television channels in desperate search of a good game, you leave him the hell alone. Take some time for yourself. Hit the salon. Hang with the girls at the mall. Rent a movie and watch it in the next room, taking small breaks to blow him kisses from afar. He'll absolutely adore you for the space.

But don't ever—EVER—try to come between a black man and his sports.

You'll never win.

My father says one of the things he most adored about my mother when they first started dating was that she loved baseball. Daddy says she spent more time watching the championship Mets (when they were a real team) on television than he did—and would get mad as hell if he tried to drag *her* away from the game. Because she appreciated the fact that he left her alone during the baseball season, she made a point of not bothering him during the football and basketball seasons.

For this sports lover, it was a match made in heaven.

Thirty-three years later, it still is.

Don't Get All Worked Up Because He Forgot Your Birthday or Buys You Cheap Gifts

Why is it that a guy can tell you the day Jackie Robinson integrated baseball, the exact number of strokes it took for Tiger Woods to win the Masters and the play-by-play description of that 1993 Knicks-Bulls playoff game when John Starks did a left-handed dunk over Michael Jordan—but they can't remember your damn birthday?

I don't know either.

Perhaps it's in the genes.

There's just no other way to explain why we're the ones who always remember the birthdays, the anniversaries, the holidays, the special occasions, the dates, places, and times of tender moments we've shared with brothers—and they haven't a clue. I mean, I used to have to call my dad once a day, every day, for two weeks before Valentine's Day to remind him to buy my mom a card and some flowers or something, because the date of February 14, the hearts, the balloons, the stupid cupids hanging up all around town—none of that stuff had any significance for him until it was absolutely too late. And I tell you, even with the daily reminders, I still almost always ended up buying her card on his behalf and leaving it somewhere for him to sign so it would at least look like he knew what was up. Ditto for her birthday, their anniversary, and any other holiday that he didn't get paid to stay home from work.

Special dates like that just don't register with them for some reason like they do for us. We can tell him from the year down to the second hand when we first made eye contact, when we shared our first kiss, when we held our first picnic together. We can tell him when his birthday is, as well as his mama's birthday and that of his first cousin on his daddy's side. And we sure as hell can't understand why he can't do the same. Remembering these special things, after all, is a symbol that we're number one in his life—that he knows these moments were important and significant in the scheme of our relationships and our lives.

So we give him hell if he forgets—act like he stole from our mama if he comes in the house without a gift on any day we deem a special occasion to be celebrated. In the doghouse he goes, with no warning, no explanations. Just to the doghouse, do not pass go, do not collect two hundred dollars.

And then the tension comes.

My father-in-law, Chikuyu, says the first time he forgot a special occasion with his then-new wife, Migozo, a chill hung over their house for a solid two weeks. He had no earthly idea what he had done wrong—just that he, at some point that month, had fallen into the bad graces of the woman he loved. She didn't speak to him unless spoken to. Her answers came in short, clipped sentences. I don't need to stress what else wasn't being done.

Then finally, she broke down and told him why she wasn't speaking to him. He had forgotten something (he didn't recall what it was when he told me this story) special, and she was letting him (not) have it. Naturally, he spent a good chunk of time trying to make it back into her good graces. Fortunately, she eventually got over it.

Those who are not married to us are not always so lucky. I have a few girlfriends who think that if a guy forgets a birthday, anniversary, Valentine's Day, or any other occasion he should automatically be dismissed. No man who truly loves them would forget something like a birthday—not if he really cared about them.

A Sistahs' Rules girl knows that's a waste of a perfectly good man.

Just because he forgets a special occasion doesn't mean he doesn't care for you. There might be other things on his mind.

I'm not saying you should accept the fact that he didn't get you those roses until February 15, or that watch until a few days after your birthday. But it's certainly not worth cutting him off over.

What you need to do is train him. There isn't a single, solitary thing you can't train a mammal to do. Hey, Pavlov did it with the dogs, didn't he?

Do what Migozo and my mom do; drop hints like a mug. Circle dates on the calendar—in bright red ink. Start talking early about what gifts you would just love to get for the holiday. Ask him what he'd like for your anniversary. My mom buys my dad Valentine's Day gifts and cards, and gives them to him on February 13. You should see how fast he runs out for his gifts now.

The point here is that you have to show him how important those days are to you. If you cut him off over it, it's not like you're going to get anything on those days anyway—so what's the point? It's a very minor thing that just isn't worth shutting him out over, especially if he's a good man in every other respect. Just ask Migozo and my mom, both of whom have been married for well over three decades.

Another thing sistahs need to stop tripping over is the quality of the gifts. I have a friend who will dismiss a brother in a heartbeat if his gift isn't up to her standard; it has to be some kind of expensive jewelry or piece of clothing or flowers in order for her to keep him around. If the guy comes back with what she considers to be a cheap trinket, out the door he goes.

Which explains why her butt has no man.

Sistahs' Rules girls know that it's not the price or quality of the gift that counts, but the thought behind it. So what if he only bought you a card; did you read the words inside it? Did it ever occur to you that that's all he had money for? The fact of the matter is that he was thinking about you—that he stood in the Mahogany section of the Hallmark store and pored over the cards until he found the one that said just how he felt about you. That's what you need to be paying attention to.

When we first started dating, my honey came up to me and pressed a red plastic heart necklace into my palm. To a non-Sistahs' Rules girl, it would have been nothing more than a stupid, cheap plastic heart. To me it was a sweet symbol of affection—a reminder that even when we weren't together, he was thinking about me. I hung that heart up on my wall the day I got it, and went to sleep with my eyes trained upon it. It made me giggle.

To this day, that red plastic heart hangs in our bedroom.

I wouldn't give up my heart for the world.

Shield Your Building from the Blaze

Eddie Murphy once joked that herpes is like luggage—something you buy once and you keep for the rest of your life. "One of these days," he lamented, sexually transmitted diseases are going to turn into super illnesses with unconquerable strains so destructive that "when we stick it in, it will explode."

It was funny as hell then—I giggled my ass off at the mere thought. Neither I, nor Eddie, nor anyone else watching that comedy sketch in the mid-eighties would ever have imagined that AIDS would ravage our community the way it has.

Indeed, the statistics are nothing to laugh at.

Consider this: According to the Centers for Disease Control, the leading cause of death among black women between ages twenty-five and forty-four in 1995 was AIDS. The statistics are sobering: 53 percent of the deaths of sistahs in 1995 were from that fatal disease.

Well above cancer.

Soaring above heart and liver disease.

Ridiculously higher than the number of sistahs who were murdered that year or died because of a stroke or diabetes.

There's a hodgepodge of explanations for this. Health care experts point to poverty, drug use, and the lack of access to health care as quick and clean explanations for why we're contracting the disease and dying at the rate we are. But the explanation is really much more simple than that: We're being too damn stupid with our bodies.

The CDC statistics are quite telling: Of the black women who died from acquired immune deficiency syndrome in 1995, 49 percent were intravenous drug users, 16 percent were the sex partners of intravenous drug users, 17 percent were the sex partners of men who contracted the disease by other risky behavior (multiple sex partners), and 17 percent contracted the disease from blood transfusions.

Basically, most of those who weren't taking drugs weren't protecting themselves—and 33 percent of them died because they were plain stupid. They lay down with men who were infected and fell for that "Come on, baby, I ain't got nothin' " line, and left some mother and father without a child, some child without a mother, some brother without a sister, some nephew without an aunt—some sistah without a sistah.

All because she didn't take two seconds out of the heat of passion to make him either wrap his penis or get up out of her bed.

This doesn't have to happen sistahs. A Sistahs' Rules girl knows that in her world, she is the most important being on this earth, and she respects the beauty that God has created— her body. She knows that it is just plain foolish to put herself at risk for the pain, suffering, and DEATH caused by one night of foolhardy play.

Sistahs, it's not worth it.

Protect yourselves.

Get smart, get tested, and be safe. Use condoms.

Besides that, why put yourself in the running for being a single mother? No matter how cute they come out, how much of a bond you have with that child, or how much you think you're ready for motherhood, it's still a bitch to raise a kid all by yourself—particularly if you're a sistah. Consider these facts: The Children's Defense Fund reported in February 1997 that every day in America, 1,744 black babies are born, 1,228 of them are born to unmarried mothers, 805 are born into poverty, 501 are born to mothers who are not high school graduates, and 404 are born to mothers younger than twenty.

And every last one of those mothers has to figure out how to feed, pamper, shelter, clothe, and love that child for at least eighteen years—in all too many cases, without the daddy around.

I don't think I need to tell you that's not cute.

Why put yourself through all of that when you can just wait until you're sure the time is right, until you're sure the man you're sleeping with is not only HIV- and AIDS-free but responsible enough to take care of his own? What's the rush, sistah?

There is none and there are no excuses. If you're grown enough to lie down with him, you're grown enough to protect yourself. Don't be stupid.

After You Get Your Swerve On, Leave Him

Congratulations! You got some.

Now get up out of his bed and go home.

That's right. Don't lie there and cuddle with him, don't have a long conversation about how good it was, don't fall asleep and expect to wake up to breakfast in bed. After about half an hour—an hour tops—get up, put your clothes on, tell him thanks for a terrific night, and head on back to the base.

Ditto for him.

If he's at your house, politely let him know that he can't spend the night. Tell him you had a terrific evening, but you've got an early day tomorrow, and he doesn't have to go home, but he's got to get the hell up out of your bed.

Trust me: It'll blow his mind.

See, brothers are used to dealing with sistahs who equate sex with love—the ones who think that sleeping with a guy gives them automatic rights to his house, his car, his relationships, his whereabouts, and his penis. Though he may really like her as a person and is happy he slept with her, she ruins it by trying to take things too fast.

To say they don't appreciate that would be the understatement of life.

No black man wants a clingy woman who turns sex into the occasion to suffocate him—to take up all his space. When she does that, she forces him to look for the opportunity to get his space back—which may not always be the best thing for the sistah.

What a brother wants is a woman who is confident and comfortable enough in her sexuality to sleep with a guy without saddling him with obligations—a woman who, after it's all over, won't be clingy and insecure and hounding him at work every five minutes, wondering where he is because she hasn't heard from him in the last hour. He wants a woman who will take it just as slow as he will, someone who knows that there is a possibility that this may lead to bigger and better things, but that sex is no guarantee that it will.

A sistah who can square her shoulders, say good night, and

walk out the door after a magnificent night of intimacy sends the message that she's just that kind of girl. You let him know that nothing is owed you—that you had a nice time, you'll be pleased if it happens again, but if it doesn't you'll get over it.

This, of course, is good for you, too—a great massage for your psyche. As you put on that coat and walk out that door, you are the one in control. You're not putting yourself out there to be thrown out by the brother—you will have said good-bye before he's had the chance to figure out if he wants you to leave or not. You will let him know that, yes, the sex was great, but you're going to determine if you want the relationship to go further.

Your butt will be in the driver's seat, your hands firmly planted on the steering wheel of this relationship—and you will feel confident that the decision on the next step will not lie solely in his hands.

My girl Felecia is a master at this. After courting a handsome stockbroker for two months, she decided to go ahead and sleep with the brother. It was fabulous, indeed, she says, but an hour after they finished and he'd fallen asleep, she got out of his bed, got dressed, put on her coat, and came on back over to thank him for a lovely evening, sealing her thanks with a sweet peck on his lips.

He pulled her back down and asked her to stay. She politely told him that she had an early-morning appointment that she couldn't be late for, kissed him again, and went on her merry way. She almost collapsed when she got out that door, because she'd enjoyed herself so much and she wanted to go for round two. But she knew that it would be best for her to go on home.

He hasn't stopped ringing her phone.

Now, it's important that when you do this, you don't walk away in a manner that you leave him wondering whether or not he, well, you know, got the job done. No matter how good they are, brothers are extremely insecure about their skills in the first few minutes after it's all over—especially with a new woman. If it was good, tell him so with sincerity—because if you walk away right after sex without doing so, he's going to think your actions mean that he was horrible and you were unpleased. He's also going to think that you are an incredibly insensitive woman for just upping and walking out and leaving him there to think about how bad he was. So step lightly.

If he was bad, well, it's on you to determine if there's room for improvement, if you could get used to it, or if you want to play ball somewhere else.

No matter the performance, though, just remember: You, sistah, are the one in control. So come strapped with your protection and your walking shoes—and watch him hang on your every move.

How to Determine He's into You and Not Just the Nookie

It's important that you understand the difference between the man who's really into you and a man who's just tolerating you. The brother who likes you will want to be around you—he will do almost anything you ask him to if he thinks he might be in it with you for the long haul. The brother who has no intention of sticking around will simply tolerate your behind until something better comes along.

Know where you stand.

The way you do that is really very simple: It's all in the dates he keeps with you.

A brother who's not really interested in a long-term relationship will do everything within his power to keep your contact short, hot, and sweet. Basically, he'll make sure that the only thing you two do is bone.

Let's face it: Given the choice between having sex with someone we don't like and sitting home with the *TV Guide* and the remote, we sistahs will almost always choose the remote. Brothers, on the other hand, would rather get some—and they'll stick around anyone who will give it to them, even if they don't really care for her that much. They have an amazing ability to tolerate people, and they will keep coming back for more if you let them. They'll simply tune you out without being really obvious about it, pulling off the one thing that we've been complaining about for centuries—being there without really being there. Unfortunately, sometimes we sistahs make it really easy for them to do that. All our man has to do is nod a few times, say "uh-huh" at the right junctures, and we're dumb enough to be happy about it. For us, it's all good until we realize he really wasn't there in the first place; for him, it's a necessary sacrifice to play you for the nookie. He regards it like he regards movie previews before the main show, like the salad before the main course—like the NBA regular season before the playoffs. He can sit through the beginning, so long as he knows for sure that the latter is well on the way.

How do you know that's what he's using you for? Well, the signals are real obvious once you take two seconds to look for them.

For instance, if you hear yourself asking him if he can meet you at the local museum at 3:00 P.M., then go with you for an early dinner, and he says, "Uh, nah, nah—I'll be busy then, but how about drinks at ten P.M.?," chances are he's trying to start the date as late as possible so that he can get to the sex quicker. Remember, he's trying to whittle down the unpleasantness of your company to the shortest possible time increments—so that you two can get right to the nookie.

But you know you have a good brother who's actually considering a long-term commitment when he willingly does things with you—things he'd never do on his own—knowing full well that there's a big, BIG chance that he won't be getting any when it's all over. He'll say yes to a date at the museum, the local theater, the mall, the ballet—hell, a movie with subtitles, if you guarantee him that you'll be doing it together. Remember: A brother isn't going to spend all that time and all that energy with someone he doesn't want to be around. He's going to search for reasons to be around you, even if it means doing something he can't stand.

How do you test it? After you've had sex with him and you think he might be interested in keeping the relationship going, invite him to do something with you that starts early in the day and will likely end with him not having the chance to initiate sex. Say you're going to the circus with your godchild in the afternoon; then afterward, you're going to drive him back home—where you will spend the night with his mom because it'll likely be too late to try to drive all the way back to your apartment. Invite him along, let him know you want him to go to the circus with you and help you drive for five hours. See if he goes for it.

If he does, girl, you might have a keeper on your hands.

If he doesn't, try again. After the third time he turns down a date that would end with no sex, you should get rid of him and move on to the next one—because he's really not all that interested in being with you. It'll hurt—but not as much as it would if you sat there and continued to get played.

It's just no fun.

Don't Compare Him to Your Last Man

It would be pretty unfair if your new man got put through the ringer because the last man dogged you. But hey, when it comes to relationships, who ever plays fair?

We're famous for holding the current beau accountable for the failings of the former. You know how it goes: The last one turned you out in the sack, but Lord if he didn't screw up in every other part of the relationship. He was irresponsible. He was lazy and unmotivated. He was a master liar and unfaithful. He didn't treat you right—and used and abused your relationship.

He stomped all over your heart and strolled away like you didn't mean a thing.

You were hurt, but you moved on; you found a new man. But he hasn't been in your life but a hot second before you start comparing him to the last fool—searching for all the mistakes and screwups the last guy made so that you can brace yourself for when the new one gets ready to take his ten-minute stroll on your feelings, too.

Don't do that.

It's called baggage—and if you carry it into your new relationship, your new man's going to immediately assess that dating you and your old ghosts is too much of a heavy burden for him to bear, and he'll step. He'll know, after all, that he won't ever be able to change what happened in your last relationship any more than you can—and he certainly won't appreciate being held accountable for the foul things somebody else did to you. All you'll be left with are bitter memories of the good one who left you, and the not-so-good one who ruined it for you.

Besides, when you spend all your time looking for signs that your new potential Brother Mr. Right is going to hurt you, you overlook all the good things that he's doing to and for you while you wait for the ball to drop on your head. You can't enjoy yourself—and you end up denying yourself the chance to make your new relationship work and be happy with him.

Why bother with all that? Sistah' Rules girls know that their past relationships are official black history—instances to learn from but never to be repeated. Now, if he's so much like the last idiot that he unmistakably possesses the same bad qualities, then yes, it could be a sign from up above that you should dump his butt. But make sure that they are indeed the same bad qualities, and not just you searching for something that's just not there.

On the flip side, you should also make a concerted effort to stop yourself from dumping your new man just because he doesn't possess some of the better qualities your last man had. For instance, if your last man sent you flowers every week and was really good in bed, don't fault the new guy if he sends you flowers only on special occasions and isn't all that great a lover. Remember, the relationship ended for a reason; the flowers and good sex obviously weren't enough for you two to keep it going. The new guy could always learn to please you sexually, and you can start giving him weekly gifts to convey the message that you'd like weekly gifts in return. What you want to make sure of is that the new one is treating you right—that he's far beyond the doormat treatment your ex was used to doling out.

My friend Keith is trying to teach that to my girl Renee. Homegirl was so used to getting dogged out by brothers that she had built this ironclad shelter around her heart. Her former boyfriends had committed a number of crimes of passion against her; some cheated, others lied—all of them hurt her so that she just couldn't bring herself to trust that any black man could possibly treat her the way a true lady should be treated.

Then came my boy Keith.

He wined and dined her. He held meaningful, intelligent conversation with her. He didn't rush her into sex, and treated her with great dignity and respect. Despite all that, she still kept bracing herself for the big let-down. If he showed up five minutes late, Renee automatically assumed that he was going to stand her up. If he wasn't home around the time that he said he would be, she would assume that he was either out with another woman, or avoiding answering the phone because he was entertaining another babe. If he mentioned another woman's name in passing, she would flip on him—assume that he wasn't being honest about seeing other women.

To his credit, Keith didn't hold it against her. He did, however, repeatedly assure Renee that he wasn't "out to get her," that she didn't have to brace herself for him to mess up because he really, really cared for her and had every honest intention of making their relationship work. He did, however, insist that Renee get counseling, so that she could work through the anger and hostility she had with the brothers who dogged her out. And get a load of this: He offered to go with her!

Now that's a good black man, y'all.

A real good one.

Girlfriends Are Everything, but They Don't Know It All

So what if your girlfriend thinks he's not all that cute?

Who cares that his "vibe" doesn't sit well with her?

What does it matter that his car, house, clothes, and tastes aren't up to par with what she's accustomed to?

Your girlfriend is neither dating nor sleeping with your potential Brother Mr. Right (at least you hope not)—you are. No matter how close you two are, no matter the number of common interests you share, your tastes in men will never be the same. She may like them tall, thin, and muscular; you may dig a guy who's not so tall and a tad more stocky. Her ideal man may be the one who drives a fancy car, makes a six-figure salary at a prestigious law firm, and comes from a family that owns a summer house on the Vineyard—but the guy you brought to her house for dinner drives a Corolla, teaches eighth-grade mathematics, and supports a family that lives in the not-so-nice section of town.

You're girls, but you're two entirely different people, and the desires and expectations you've each set for your mates will hardly ever jibe. So when she looks him up and down and turns up her nose when she sees the Corolla in the driveway, pull her aside and check her. When it comes down to decisions like whether you'll date him despite the fact that he doesn't look like Grant Hill or have his NBA money, you have to remember that he's your man, not hers.

That's not to say that her opinions shouldn't be taken into account when you're making important relationship decisions. She's your girlfriend, and sistahs know that there's nothing like a good girlfriend with a strong shoulder and a comforting word. They're there to giggle, gossip, shop, and dream with you, worry, struggle, pray, and cry with you, and, at the end of the day, hand over the Kleenex when he's gone and messed things up. Simply, she's everything to you.

When your in-love-but-blind behind can't see that he's just no damn good, she's going to tell you about it. She's equipped with a special radar—a sixth sense that can spot a trifling Negro quicker than the bat of an eyelash. She's good at—and damn sure will be—pointing it out.

But she's not a mind reader, she doesn't know everything about everybody, and she certainly isn't perfect. Above all, her tolerance levels are not always going to be in lockstep with yours. Where she would immediately dismiss a man who cheated on her once, you might be the type who would get over the fling and work at making the relationship last.

You also have to recognize that when girlfriend tells you he's no good for you, or that he takes up too much of your time and you don't need him, she may be saying that because she doesn't have a potential Brother Mr. Right of her own. Remember: Misery just loves some company—and sister girl may subconsciously be giving you bad advice because she doesn't want him to cut into the quality time she shares with you.

Your job is to flesh out her advice, swallow it with a grain of salt, take your own feelings into consideration, weigh your options, and make the relationship decisions for yourself by yourself. Her job is to sit back and let you stumble through your mistakes and be there for you when you fall—the way a true friend would.

So that your sistahs know their role in your relationships, here's a short, four-item tip sheet you can give them for their conduct. I call it the "Know Your Place, Girlfriend" list.

Stick to Your Own Wish List

Sistahs' Rules girls know what they want. The wish list is clear, they've written it out, made changes, agreed to a few concessions and checked it twice, by themselves. You, girlfriend, have no power to make amendments to it—so don't go there. Jada used this one to put Jennifer in check when Jennifer tried to tell Jada that her man wasn't good enough for her. Truth be told, he fit Jada's wish list just fine; he was sweet, intelligent, trustworthy, and he treated her right—what Jada asked for in her wish list. Jennifer's wish list, obviously, was more involved and a lot more superficial—and Jada's man just wasn't up to snuff. Jada quickly pointed out that they were operating from two different pages, and advised Jennifer that she would be wise to stick to her own list when she got her own man. No more problems out of Jennifer.

Respect My Tolerance Levels

No two women are the same; this much is obvious. What one sistah can take, the other may not be able to stomach for a single minute. But one is no better than the other, and you, if you are a true friend, must let her decide when enough is enough— without giving her grief for not doing it the way you would have done it. Like with Monica. She found out the hard way that her man was cheating on her; just as she, her boyfriend Edward, and her girlfriends Shawn and Denise were about to be seated for dinner, a woman strolled up to Edward, asked him who Monica was, and then slapped him in the face when he didn't answer fast enough. Didn't take a rocket scientist to figure out that Edward had a little somethin' going on the side. Shawn and Denise knew Monica was going to drop his butt right there in the restaurant, but she didn't. Monica went on as if nothing had happened and saved her confrontation with Edward for later. They talked it out and Monica ended up staying with her cheatin' man. Shawn and Denise couldn't believe it and told her if that was their man, they would have kicked him to the curb immediately. But Monica didn't think that was worth firing Edward; she wanted to work it out. That was her prerogative. Shawn and Denise, as her girlfriends, had no other choice but to respect that.

Remember That Penis Envy Is Not Cute

A note to the girlfriends who don't have men: Leave the blocking to the football players. Just because you don't have one doesn't mean your girl can't have one. She knows that she isn't spending as much quality time with you, but that doesn't mean you are less important in her heart. Coupling up is what grown-ups do—and you have to make sure that you're mature enough to handle the fact that she's building a grown-up relationship, and do whatever it is that you can do to support the relationship, rather than sabotage it. Maia got a reputation among her girl-friends for trying to bust up couples. The funny thing was that she didn't realize what she was doing; Maia had convinced her-self that she was simply being frank with her girlfriends about their men and their trifling ways. One of my girls, Yvette, sat her down one day and broke it down for her, though, because she got tired of Maia's meddling. Maia was ticked, but she got over it. And sure as the day is long, when that girl found herself a man, she didn't have the time on her hands to intertwine herself into our affairs. All of us were better off for it.

Be There for Me

No, your girlfriend didn't listen to you and stayed with that foolish man, only to get her feelings hurt—just like you pre-dicted. That's no reason for dogging her out with a running commentary on "I Told You So." What she needs right now is for you to simply listen. That's all, just listen. That's the most girlfriend could possibly expect from you. Take, for instance, the time when Verna's longtime boyfriend told her that he was moving in with another woman. Verna's girl Sharon had long told her that he was no good, and Verna knew it—but she stayed with him anyway. When Patrick moved in with the other woman, Verna was heartbroken beyond belief. The last thing she needed was for Sharon to get in her face, talking about "See?

What did I tell you?" To her credit, Sharon came over to Verna's with a box of tissues, a couple of videos, and some old records, and lent her ear and shoulder to her best girlfriend until her tears dried up.

Four things—that's all a true girlfriend's responsible for in her sistah's relationship. You'd be amazed how much luggage is removed from a relationship between a man and woman when girlfriend sticks to the guidelines.

Of course, you have to be wary of the clingers—the women who will stick around you for the sake of clinging on to your man. Oh, come on now—you know it happens. She worms her way into your home, sucks up to you and your man; then the minute you turn around, she strikes out like a prowling cobra lunging for its prey. She's hard to recognize; she's friendly, she goes shopping with you, she cooks for you and your man, and she proclaims both you and he are her closest friends. Her horns don't show.

You won't know what hit you until it's too late.

Dorothy didn't. She had a friend, Bridgette, with whom she hung out regularly. They did everything together, and eventually became so close that Bridgette had taken to calling Dorothy's mother "Mom." Bridgette also took a hankering to convincing Dorothy to visit her boyfriend's house with her—just to hang out. Dorothy didn't realize it, but Bridgette was worming her way into Dorothy and Anthony's relationship. Funny thing:

Bridgette set it up so that Anthony looked like he was cheating on Dorothy. Of course, Dorothy, who has no tolerance for men who cheat, quit Anthony. Bridgette was all too happy to take her place. Now she has Anthony's baby.

Go figure.

I'd say kill her, but Dorothy would go to jail for that and then what use would she be to anybody?

No, really—Dorothy just took it as a learning experience and moved on. Luckily, she was surrounded by a few more genuine girlfriends who had no problem helping her through the hard time.

That's, after all, what friends are for.

The final word: If you find yourself questioning the advice of your girlfriend, you can always turn to Mama—'cause she'll never steer her baby wrong.

Nuff said.

Be His Homie

You want to be more than a screw-buddy with him? Try being his friend, why don't you?

Oh, you'll be amazed how quick a brother will put you at the top of his "Got to Have Her" list once he feels comfortable enough to open up to you.

See, it's a rarity that they get to do that with anyone—even their boys. In fact, brothers' relationships with brothers are as peculiar and as complex as Michael Jackson and his skin: we sistahs look at both of them in awe and wonder how in the hell it hasn't sloughed off after years of obviously unhealthy treatment.

They're just nothing like the friendships we

build with our sistahs: We talk about anything under the sun—sex, relationships, insecurities, love, work, money, and weaknesses. We're comfortable sitting next to each other on the couch and sharing our innermost emotions; it's a woman's way.

When they get together with their boys, they'll talk about everything under the sun all right—everything except their true feelings. With their boys, they keep up this front like they're strong mentally, physically, and emotionally all day, every day— even though during the course of their 24-7, they experience just as many problems, want just as much understanding, and need just as many shoulders to lean on as we look for when we run to our sistahs for support.

Showing weakness and vulnerability to the fellas is not an option.

So if his love interest is making more money than he is and he's upset about it, or she's smarter than he is and he can't handle that? His boy will never know.

If another brother at work keeps getting the promotions and props he thinks he deserves and he's jealous of him? Oh, hell no—he'll never tell his friend.

If he really, really likes this sistah and thinks she might be the one? His homie won't find out about it until he sees the ring on the chick's finger or he gets the wedding invitation in the mail.

A brother wants and needs to make it seem like he's always got the upper hand in the relationships, the upper hand at work—the upper hand at everything, because that makes him out to be the strong black man. Society has him all turned around on his place in this world; he's supposed to be strong because he's a man—but every day he keeps being told or shown in some kind of foul way that because he's black, he's not really a man. That means that even with his boys, the ones that he talks sports with, the ones that he sips beer at the bar with and macks the women with are not necessarily going to know that he's bothered by anything, that something has him hurting.

Where do you stand in all of this? You're supposed to be the one who can break through that tough-guy shell—make him feel like he can trust you with the feelings he spends so much time hiding from everyone else. That's, after all, what friendship is all about: Comfort level. You have to learn how to make him comfortable with you.

It's not easy, but it can be done.

A good start would be to avoid being overly critical and judgmental. An even better one would be to avoid pushing him into telling you how he feels. You're not Rolanda, and he's not on the stage of a talk show willing to tell all of America his business. He's a brother and, above all else, a man. His nature is to flex muscles, not show vulnerability. If you constantly nag him to tell you how he feels, he'll treat you like you're a nag.

Create an environment where he can reveal to you that he's got a problem, and you are going to listen to it, absorb it, give him a hug, and leave it alone; an environment where he can drop it, feel like he's got something off his chest, and feel comfortable that he's not going to be any less of a man for it. For instance, if he's a little short on cash and he knows that you wanted to go someplace special, he should be able to tell you he's a little light in the pocket—without you making a big deal about it. If his ex-wife is putting him through the ringer over their kid, or plain giving him a hard time, he should be able to tell you she's driving him crazy, without you screaming, yelling, and telling him, "Go get your coat—let's go burn her house down!"

Just listen. If he asks for advice, give it. If he doesn't, don't offer it, because chances are, he's not looking for solutions—he's just looking for a sympathetic ear. The woman who's able to negotiate that delicate balance is the one who's going to make him feel like he has someone in his corner—the one he's most likely to want in his life.

You could also get serious "She's a Keeper" points if you make having fun with him just as important as making love to him. Don't make it all about romance all of the time. You want him to know that a relationship with you isn't always about work—that there are some fun times mixed up in there, too. Instead of suggesting a romantic dinner by candlelight, put on your boots and go hiking with him. Rather than plan that romantic picnic for Sunday, take him out to the tennis court and show him a thing or five. Go to the gym with him, exercise together—join the bowling league or throw a slamming party and invite all of your friends to dance the night away with you both.

Let loose and have some fun with the man. Make him want to be around you for more than just sex. When he realizes he's got a good listener on his hands, one who isn't afraid to let her braids down, oh—you're in there, sistah.

In there.

Get to Know His Mama, Get to Know Him

My mother-in-law said it best when she offered this tidbit: "Know where he's coming from, because eventually, he's going to go right back to it."

It's quite logical, really—and our own mothers have practiced this throughout the ages. Remember when you were little, and your mama didn't let you go over to your little friend's house but once because she'd seen it and it was nasty and Mrs. So and So, your friend's mama, didn't have any manners and her attitude was really funky? Perhaps you didn't quite understand right at that moment why your mother didn't want you over there or hanging with your friend, but as time passed, you realized that you didn't like hanging with her anyway because she was just like her mama—a little nasty, a little short on the manners, and definitely the bearer of funky attitudes.

You quickly surmised that she got that from her mama.

See, they're almost always one and the same—mothers and kids. The things you like and dislike, the way you carry yourself, the values you hold dear—your entire way of life—is rooted in the way you were brought up. The way things went down in your house when you were little, you consider absolutely normal, because that was your life and the way your parents set it up for you.

It's no different for black men.

The single most important woman in a black man's life next to his wife is his mother. He has a special bond with his mama, because she's the one who took special care to nurture him, shelter him, and protect him from a harsh society that seems always to stand ready to put men of color through all sorts of hell. She's the one who shielded her own young black males the best she could—the one who, as she was raising her daughter, was busy loving and protecting her son. If nothing went drastically wrong in their relationship, he holds her dear because of that special bond.

He's going to look for a sistah who can best fulfill two roles: that of a mate and, to some extent, that of his mama. He doesn't want to marry his mother, of course—but he does admire her characteristics and looks to see that at least some of them are present in the mate he's going to spend the rest of his life with. Likewise, the way his mother keeps house, the values and expectations she lives by, the attitude she takes with the world are likely the same that your man will have. Hey, he had to get them from somewhere—and almost every time, they came from mommy.

So if you want to know where he's going, check out where—more specifically, whom—he came from. It'll be revealing.

I've devised for you some simple signs to heed when you meet his mama—some telltale signals that should reveal to you what kind of man you have on your hands. Remember that none of it is cut-and-dried; but it will certainly help you out just a little bit in understanding him better and recognizing what kind of characteristics he's looking for in a mate.

The "Angela Davis Is My Hero" Mama

She's a lot of fun—an interesting character to behold. You go to her house and everything there is in the shape of the motherland—down to the coasters. She wouldn't put chemical products in her hair unless someone strapped her down and knocked her out—but her strength and will would allow her to wake up and kick the products out of your hand anyway. Her TV channels pick up only *Like It Is* and *Positively Black,* she's a strict vegetarian, and she thinks that Malcolm X, Angela Davis, and

Huey Newton were prophets sent to black people from on high. She will not want her baby dating or marrying a woman who thinks Eldridge Cleaver is the brand name for a new line of knives. Your man may not be exactly like his mama, but you can bet that he will be politically conscious, that he's going to take a special interest in knowing, caring about, and helping his people, and that he will give up his time to the woman who is willing to do the same. The red flag here is that his mother could assume from one look at your weave and your light skin that you're not black enough—so you may be forced to prove it at some point. But if you can hang, you have nothing to worry about here.

The "Mean as Hell" Mama

She's not the nicest person in the world. She's unemotional. She doesn't hug her son, she clips conversations short, and she's unmoved by any turn of events—whether it be happy or sad. Her kids probably grew up thinking their middle names were "dumb ass," being overly criticized, and having their needs swept behind her own constantly. She may even be mean in an acerbically funny sense—really sarcastic and harsh. She can break her kids down in the bat of an eyelash, and treats all who come in contact with her like they're hecklers at one of her stand-up performances. You may have trouble on your hands, sistah—because this brother may be just like his mama.

What you need to look out for here is whether he's just like his mama or if he shuns her. If he takes after her, he, too, may be mean and unemotional, because he never got that kind of special feeling from the one woman in his life who was supposed to show him that emotional love. He also may not be very good with kids, because he may take cues from his mother on how to raise them—in a not-so-loving environment—and he may make you and yours the brunt of sarcastic, critical jokes that are cute at first, but a pain in the butt when they keep coming. If he shuns the way his mother treated him, he may well expect his woman to be the complete opposite of the unemotional, taxing woman his mother is. Look out for the signs.

The "Super-Nice" Mom

She's the black version of June Cleaver. In fact, she'd put old June to shame. She bakes cookies, she washes his clothes, cooks for and cleans up after him when he's around; she babies him to no end—and he, like a little kitten being stroked by his master, loves every minute of it. There's nothing wrong with this; that's what mommies are supposed to be for. But chances are that if he expects you to follow in her footsteps, he may have a few expectations that just don't jibe with the nineties woman you're trying to be. He'll raise an eyebrow when he walks past the dirty dishes, and you'll wonder if there's something in his eye. He'll keep telling you how much bleach he likes in his whites, and you'll continually wonder what you're supposed to do with that tidbit of information. You may catch him at the kitchen table every once in a while, sitting in front of the plate with a fork and knife in his hand. No need to fear—you can deal with this in a number of ways; you can let him know up front that you're neither his mama nor his maid, and that cooking, cleaning, and other household responsibilities are to be shared; or you can do all of it and like it. I'm not saying either one is better than the other; you just have to choose which is right for you—and make it clear where you stand.

The "Broke Down and Lonely" Mama

She doesn't have a man in her life, never had a decent one around, and thinks that most black men are nothing but trifling dogs who don't deserve a woman's time of day. You walk into her house and it becomes painfully obvious that the only thing Ms. Lady has working for her is her heat—and that's only a few months out of the year. She has no job, no prospects, no self-respect, no couch, and no clue. Of her son, you should be careful. Not to say that the products of the poor don't know how to act, but a child who is raised to think men are crap will likely think he's worthless, too. Moreover, he may have no clue what it means to be a responsible man if the woman who raised him wasn't responsible either and the most reliable man in his childhood was the mailman. You'll look at him and wonder how he made it out in one piece, still able to function in the world—and hope like hell that he figured it out somewhere else. The good thing about this is that he's probably a survivor who, because his mama wasn't giving it to him, found out how to get what he needed on his own. His expectations from women may also be a little low, so he's basically a blank slate who can be really easy to please if you break the trend that his mother set for him when he was a kid.

The "Smothering Blanket" Mama

She is, perhaps, the hardest to deal with because she's going to make a point of being all up in your business just when you don't need her to be. She gives her son about as much breathing room as a plastic bag tied over his head: absolutely none. She goes out of her way to pick and nag and tell her son what to do and how to do it—and tells him off if he strays from the way she's set. She makes it so that he can't make a move without her say-so—or he suffers the consequences. She's the epitome of the nagging mother-in-law. You are almost guaranteed that there will be times when you'll be just shy of killing her or divorcing your man, because he will likely take her side whenever forced to choose between you and her. She's his mama; you can't usurp that, no matter how hard you try. If by some act of weird, cosmic force he disowns her, well then, you have nothing to worry about. But you will have to live with the guilt of dividing him from his family. Either way, you don't win. Some folks are able to live with one of the alternatives; you have to decide what your tolerance level is, and take it from there—because I guarantee you, sistah, she will work your nerves to no end.

The perfect mama would be the one who possesses each of these characteristics—a well-grounded sistah who respects herself, is strict but not suffocating, treats her son well and defends her baby to the end. She's the one who will appreciate you for who you are, because she knows you're the one her baby wants. She'll not step in the middle of your relationship, and she'll defend and support your union—in the interest of having a happy, healthy couple in her life.

Her son will reflect that and bring it on home to you.

But this isn't a perfect world, and even mamas have baggage. Just make sure you don't end up carrying it. Get to know his mama, and you'll know just how heavy it is.

Don't Mention the "M" Word for at Least Twelve Months

For a brother, the fear incited by Freddy Krueger, Blackula, and Lamont's Aunt Esther combined can't touch that evoked at the premature mentioning of—pregnant pause—the "M" word.

I mean, the mere hint of marriage makes brothers bolt upright in their beds in the middle of the night—you must set buckets of cold ice and washrags next to the Sealy to deal with the simultaneous hot flashes and cold sweats they suffer after the matrimonial nightmares haunt their sleep. They just can't deal with the idea of the old ball-and-chain unless they're absolutely, positively, 100 percent, without a shadow of a doubt readier than a mug—and no amount of your hinting, tearfully begging, pleading, or bribing is going to bring them around any quicker.

The issue surrounding this paranoia can be summed up in a single saying:

The only thing better than poontang is new poontang.

Basically, no matter how good you are, no matter how sweet you treat him, no matter how strong the relationship—in the back of his mind, he's going to almost always figure that there's some woman out there who might be even better.

Call it the grass-is-always-greener syndrome.

Factor into that his hesitancy and outright unwillingness to exchange his freedom to ho stroll for a life of "yes, dear," kids, and family responsibility, and you've got yourself the reason why your man—no matter how sane and rational he might appear to be—will completely lose his mind when you mention that, that—word in his presence.

Which is exactly why you shouldn't even think of saying the words *marriage, ceremony, ring,* or *"I do"* at anytime, anywhere until you've been in a committed relationship with him for at least a year. After twelve months, you guys should pretty much know everything about each other—or at least enough to tell if a lifetime together could be a possibility.

Anything less than that and you're liable to give the poor brother a heart attack.

You want that time to figure out if he's good enough for you, anyway. Is he good to you? Do you think he would be a good father to your kids? Can you trust him? Does he respect you? Is he a good lover? Is he a good provider? Does he make you happy? This is, after all, the man with whom you're going to stand before God and declare to love, honor, and cherish and all that good stuff for the rest of your life. This is nothing to rush for you either.

You, of course, don't want to waste a whole lot of time with a guy who has no intention of getting married—if that's what you're looking for. Within the first three months, you should have that little cursory probing session where you two discuss each other's intentions for the future—you know, "So? How many kids do you want? What age would you like to see yourself married? Do you even believe in marriage?" This won't bother him, so long as you don't get deep with it. He's not stupid; he knows that in the back of your mind, you're sizing him up as husband material. But don't get deep with it, or he might go running.

That means that you can't walk past the jewelry store, then pull him by the coattail and tell him that you prefer a two-carat pear-shaped diamond over a six-point baguette.

That means you don't pull out your worn edition of *Jumping the Broom* every time he's around and mark it up with red ink—then ask him how he'd like his ceremony to be conducted.

That means you don't ask him for the travel agent's name so that you can start planning the honeymoon.

Or else he's outta there.

After the year of committed relationship with him—that means a year from the day you two decided to date exclusively, not from the date that you first saw him in the parking lot at the grocery store—you should casually strike up the "intentions" conversation—the one where you feel him out on the marriage thing. If he's clearly not with it, don't push him—he will come around if he's serious about you and your relationship.

A special note about parents: You have to take him to Mom and Dad's house eventually; your parents have every right to know who their baby's seeing, you have to get the all-important verdict from your mother, and he should know about your family and acquaint himself with them. But know that it's a minefield to sit him down at the Thanksgiving table—because somebody's bound to ask you both when you're going to get hitched. I mean, moms are like that; the day you got your college diploma, your mother said, "Oh, baby, I'm so happy! You graduated from college—now when you getting married?" They want to see their kid walk down the aisle and they want the grandparents title. They will not stand by and let you tread lightly on that—particularly if you bring a gentleman friend to the house. They have no couth. So make sure you sit him down before you take him there and warn him that nothing they say about marriage is to be taken seriously, and that you had nothing to do with it if they do, indeed, ask him his intentions. This way, he won't choke on his turkey and candied yams.

If by the third year, though, he hasn't initiated an "intentions" conversation, and he's still turning deep shades of purple when you start one up, then you need to rethink whether he's really serious about your relationship—because after three years, both of you should know whether the other is "the one" by now. Sitting in the relationship for a few years more isn't going to prove anything; it'll simply ensure him more stalling time. Besides, you don't want to turn around seven years into this relationship and still be dating him and have no ring on your finger, because by then, you'll never want to leave. You'll figure, "Hey, I spent seven good years of my life in a relationship with this man, and I'll be damned if I'm going to give him up now." Then, the next thing you know, you've never married him—just been with him forever.

That's not good enough, sistah.

I have a girlfriend who's been dating her man for eleven years now—and she's absolutely miserable. Their relationship is perfectly fine, mind you. But her peace of mind is ridiculously shot because she can't convince her boyfriend to marry her. He's afraid that if he does get married, he won't be able to further his career like he wants to. She's afraid that if she lets him go after all these years, she'll never find another guy because she's in her late thirties and all the good ones that age are already taken.

Poor thing.

Personally, I'd leave his butt. Sistahs' Rules girls know about the bus—and how often it can come along if you give it a route. She, however, feels like she's stuck.

Don't go out like that, girl. Plan it wisely, and make sure that both of you are ready for the "M" thing. Rushing into it won't help matters, and neither will sitting around waiting for him to decide what he's going to do. Be like a jogger running a marathon; do it at a steady pace, speed up when the energy is right and slow it down when you need to build it up.

You can't win every time, but you can always make sure you cross that finish line—some way, somehow. Hopefully, the two of you can do it together, without any help from Freddy, the Count, or Aunt Esther.

Give Him the Option of Commitment

Oh, we're good for telling a brother to commit or step. Then, through tear-filled eyes, we watch him walk right out the door and into the arms of some other woman—and run and tell our girlfriends, mothers, therapists, *Essence* and *Oprah* that black men are afraid of settling down.

For the record, most African-American men are not afraid of what I call the "Big C"—commitment. Despite what statistics, analysts, and the five o'clock news lead you to believe, black men love black women, they like the concept of marriage—so long as it's with the right lady—and they adore being fathers.

It's ultimatums that send them out of our lives screaming like banshees.

I can't blame them for hollering.

A person—man or woman—needs choices to remain stable. You go to several shoe stores in search of the perfect pair of brown suede pumps because you know that even though you really, really liked the ones in Macy's, Saks just might have some that you'll like even better. You go to Pathmark instead of the corner bodega because at the grocery store you can choose between Ball Park franks, Nathan's long and thin hot dogs, or No Frills, rather than being forced to buy the one no-named brand stocked in the corner store. You appreciate the options, because without them, you either buy the product that you really don't want, or you do without it because it's not what you like.

The same thing applies to men and relationships. When a woman takes away a man's choices, he lashes out—mainly because he feels like he's being suckered into making a deal that he's not so sure he wants to make. In an instant, his freedom is taken away—not by his own choice, but by a woman who's basically told him to either put his mental and physical desires for other women on immediate lockdown or walk away from a relationship that he may have just started really digging.

Shackles or freedom. Freedom, shackles.

For a guy, it's not a hard decision. Try not to inhale while you're watching his smoke.

How do you keep him from running? Give him options— two is all you need. Tell him he can either commit to the relationship—just the two of you working toward a serious one-on-one gig—or he can continue to date other women—with the understanding that you, too, will date other men—while you two figure out if a long-term relationship together is workable.

If you get the Big C right off the bat, then you're the woman. Congratulations, girl, because you've worked a mojo on him so well that he wants to date you and only you. And we all know that exclusivity is a beautiful thing when it's done with the one you love.

But ninety-nine out of one hundred times, brotherman is going to tell you he's really, really into Option No. 2—the one where he gets to have his cake and eat it, too.

Hear me out, sistahs.

He knows that Option No. 1 means the games are over, no more playtime—really serious business. He also knows that Option No. 2 offers a tad bit more flexibility—a chance to get to know a sistah better while he gets all that playing out of his system. When extended the courtesy of the latter option, he'll appreciate that you recognize he's just not ready for commitment and are willing to see if you two are indeed right for each other before you ask him to burn the little black book.

The funny thing about this is that his picking Option No. 2 will probably get him to commit quicker than any ultimatum trip you lay on him. That's because he'll be extremely bothered by the fine print in Option No. 2—the one that says you, my dear sistah, get to play the field, too. Brothers' egos are entirely too large for them to allow their main squeeze to be shared with other brothers. They want that cake all to themselves, because they're just selfish like that.

My girl Regina can attest to this one. She told her guy pal Scott after three months of dating that she was ready for a committed relationship with him, but she didn't want to rush him into anything. Then she laid out the options. He, without hesitation, picked No. 2. Two weeks later, while he was at her house, Regina's phone rang several times—and each ring was met by the answering machine. Scott demanded to know why Regina wasn't answering the phone or listening to the messages. "You're afraid that it might be one of your little boyfriends calling here, and you don't want me to hear it," he accused.

Regina simply responded by telling him that what was on her answering machine and on the other end of her phone was none of his concern—because he was not officially her man. What she did and who she did it with on her own time were her business.

Scott didn't like it, but what choice did he have? He was the one who chose Option No. 2, fine print and all.

Needless to say, two weeks later, *he* was asking for a committed relationship from *her*!

Works every time.

Truth be told, when that happens, you should tell him that you want—and need—to stick to Option No. 2 anyway—because this way, you get to evaluate whether your potential Brother Mr. Right is the one you really want. That he wanted to play the field in the first place should have told you that he may not have been as serious about your relationship as you thought he was. You can't let his ultimatum make you rush into anything, without evaluating some choices for yourself. After all, a Sistahs' Rules girl knows that if this one doesn't work out, there are about twenty more where he came from—and if you stick to your rules, you'll get the pick of the potential Brother Mr. Right litter.

Then sit back and watch him eat your smoke.

Whether you two end up rolling with Option No. 1 or Option No. 2, you need to set some boundaries, some standards—draw some lines in the sand. If you two decide to go for the committed, one-on-one relationship, make sure he's clear on this: The Big C means a one-on-one relationship, not one-on-three. A committed relationship is built on trust and loyalty. You've got to know that this person has your back 24-7, not just when he feels like it. If either of you can't stick to that basic tenet, then that person has to be honest and let the other person know it before he/she walks out the door.

If the two of you choose Option No. 2, well then, you both have to make sure that you are completely comfortable with knowing that the other is going to be suiting up and playing the field. What you or he does outside of your couple time is neither one of you all's business. If he can't go out with you on Saturday because he has other plans, don't ask questions. But make sure that he knows you're suiting up to play the field, too. It would also be wise for you two to agree to how much quality time you will be spending with each other—so that you don't lose each other during the game.

Above all else, you need to make sure that you both are clear on whether your relationship will remain monogamous, or if you two get to have sexual relations with other people. In this day and age, I wouldn't go for that. The ideal Option No. 2 is a couple that is a step away from serious, sleeps only with one another but goes out occasionally with other people just to get that playing out of the system.

Got it? Now let's play Big C ball.

HOW TO KEEP A GOOD BLACK MAN

Give Him Three Months After He Commits to Tie Up Loose Ends

So you're having a nice candlelight dinner at your Brother Mr. Right's house, right? Will Downing is purring from the stereo speakers—you're looking into each other's eyes. Your once-lively conversation is now sweet whispers of adoration. You're both thinking it's time for dessert—but not the kind that comes on a plate.

And then, louder than a southern farm rooster's five o'clock crow, the ringing phone pierces your perfect intimate moment.

Brother strolls over to the phone, picks it up, says "Hello?" real normal-like, then starts talking real low, real polite, and real clipped, like "Yes, how are you this evening? Um, no, this is not a good time but let's discuss it tomorrow. Okay . . . same here. Okay, good night." Then, without your even asking, he comes back over to the table, tells you that that was his boy Jerome, and "Oh, by the way, where were we?"

You're not stupid; you're a Sistahs' Rules girl—and you know exactly what's up. You know that Jerome would have gotten a "What up, man? Chillin'. My baby's here—let me get with you tomorrow. Peace"—not the strictly business voice.

He's just activated your "Hoochie Alarm."

Whatever you do, don't trip! If your Brother Mr. Right is serious about your commitment to each other, then she's nothing more than a loose end—unfinished business that he hasn't dealt with just yet. Remember: Your Brother Mr. Right is an eligible and dynamic bachelor—regardless of the fact that he's agreed to commitment with you—because he has no ring on his finger. Every man is a player, and you can bet your last dollar that he had a few chippies lined up in that little black book of his before he decided he wanted to settle down into an exclusive relationship with you. They will not disappear that easily. There were women before you who probably thought they were the ones headed for the commitment, and there will be women after you who will, too, if you don't play your cards right.

So let's use this phone call as an opportunity, shall we? She—or they, for that matter—will be perfect measuring sticks by which you will gauge his seriousness to the Big C. Let them dial the digits, then watch him shuffle for the first four months of your newfound relationship. If at the beginning of the fifth month—that's the amount of time it should take to know if you're really in a serious relationship or not—the calling and other telltale signs of women on the prowl persist, casually ask him if his other suitors know he's in an exclusive relationship.

If he says, "Yes, darling, I've told them about you," then you need to figure out if he's telling the truth. He really could have been talking to Jerome, or the woman that called the house looking for him really might just be an old friend of his that just happens to be a woman. It's up to you to figure it out. Tell him that when Jerome calls, it's okay to talk to him. Tell him that you want to meet all his friends—Ms. She's Just a Friend, in particular—and then check all of them out. Make your presence known, in a nice, subtle way. If he's truly committed, he won't have a problem with it—and you'll know that you are, indeed, the woman.

But if you're seeing telltale signs that there might be others—like numbers on little pieces of crinkled-up paper keep showing up around his apartment, or the woman that you both ran into at the restaurant looked a tad too undone by the sight of you two together—then he's lying. If you have concrete evidence of this in hand, remind him of the commitment that you made to each other, let him know that the top of that agreement was that there would be no more playing the field, then throw him off your court. It's going to hurt knowing that your relationship didn't work, but it'll hurt even more if later on down the road you find out the chippies have more clout with him than you.

If he says that he kinda told his prior suitors about you "but not really," then here's what you do: Encourage him to be honest with the others if he's really serious about that love jones thang you two have going. Then, give him three months to kick them all to the curb. If he respects you and himself, and he's truly interested in building a healthy, loving, trusting relationship with you, then by the end of that three-month deadline, every man, woman, child, and other creature that breathes and thinks and knows your Brother Mr. Right should know that you and he are an item and that you play important roles in each other's lives.

That means that when his phone rings, your Brother Mr. Right greets the person by name, tells her/him that he's in the middle of dinner with you, his girlfriend, and that they will have to talk another time.

It means that when you go out in public and run into one of his old love interests or Ms. She's Just a Friend, he introduces you as his girlfriend.

It even means that he'll let you answer his phone.

No more crinkled papers, no more hang-ups, no late-night phone calls or dirty looks from the gals—the simple signs of a trusting relationship.

My girlfriend Caryl did this with her guy. A handsome devil with a line of beautiful women waiting to make him their own, Henry decided after a few months of dating that he wanted Caryl to be the one he made the commitment with. Still, it took a little longer than Caryl wanted it to for him to let the others in on that tidbit of information. So she let him know one night that he and she would be best served if he hipped them to the fact that he's off the market—and then sat back and secretly gave him three months to spread the word.

By the end of the three months, everyone knew Caryl was the queen of Henry's heart. And to show that he was indeed serious about their relationship, Henry gave Caryl the keys to his house, phone-answering privileges, and access to his E-mail account.

I don't think there's any doubt that this brother has nothing to hide; E-mail accounts are nothing to sneeze at.

Caryl, of course, is loving every minute of her royal treatment.

Make Your Past Relationships Official Black History

Do not tell your new man about that stupid argument you had with your last boyfriend, and how you made him feel really dumb once you were able to prove to him that you were right. Your new Brother Mr. Right will not be thinking about your reasoning prowess; he will be thinking about the fact that you slept with another man.

Do not tell your new guy about how happy you are that he took you on vacation to Cozumel and how he's so much better than your last man because he never thought to take you away to special places like Mexico. Your new Brother Mr. Right will not be basking in the glory of one-upping the last man; he will be thinking about the fact that you slept with another man.

Do not tell your current boyfriend that he dresses nicer, acts better, and is generally an all-round better guy than the last man. Your new Brother Mr. Right will not be impressed that he's better than your ex.

That's right—you guessed it. The only think he will take from that is that you slept with another guy.

Never, under any circumstances, should he be put in a position to think about what you've done with other men in the past—men just can't handle that truth. Sure, he knows that you weren't delivered to him in one of those lacy white dresses—the kind that, in other cultures, he would hold up to the cheering crowd that's gathered outside your balcony on your wedding night to assure that he's the one who deflowered you. But he doesn't need all the gory details, and he certainly doesn't want to think about them.

He wants his woman to have skills in the bed—but he doesn't want to know how you got there. He wants to know your favorite positions and he wants you to do interesting things while you two are making love—but he definitely doesn't want to know how you came up with the idea, how you got to it, and who you got to it with. He wants to know that you love the way he smells, but he doesn't want to be told it reminds you of some other man.

No man—whether he be black or white—likes to imagine the passion and pleasure his mate got from somebody else. Simply, it bothers the hell out of him to have to recognize that he wasn't the first. Of course, that's deeply rooted in his own insecurities. No matter how well you treat him, how many times you tell him you love him, how much you adore him, how well he performs—he's always going to wonder if he's measuring up to the last guy.

He's also more liable to think that your mind is somewhere else—that the only reason you keep bringing up the other brothers is because you never wanted to leave them in the first place. He'll think he's nothing but a way station until you can make it back to old boy.

You don't want to take him there, because it always leads to problems. Big problems.

My girl Sherrie's trying to rectify the situation with her fiancé as you read this. When she started dating Cedric, she knew right off that he was the one she wanted to spend the rest of her life with. He felt the same. She immediately assessed that there was nothing Cedric shouldn't know about her life; she felt perfectly comfortable telling him everything about her past— including who her old boyfriends were. She gave him details, y'all; told him how many there were, what their names were, where they were from, and what kinds of careers they were pursuing or holding. Just everything. And Cedric's haunted her with the information ever since. He looks for inconsistencies in her stories. He becomes retaliatory and, out of nowhere, brings up tidbits of information that she could do without—like how one of his old girlfriends had a fancy for French lingerie. When he sees her ex-boyfriends—a few of them are entertainers, so they show up occasionally in movies, videos, and commercials, etc.—he gets mad and it takes him hours to recover and act right. Sherrie finds herself constantly reminding Cedric that she loves him and him only—and that her past boyfriends are black history; never to be repeated. He shouldn't, she insists, feel weird about guys she's dated in the past, because none of them have anything to do with her relationship with him.

Cedric's gotten a little better lately, but he still finds occasion to bring the issue up every now and then. Sherrie readily admits that if she had it to do all over again, she wouldn't dare give Cedric detailed information on any of her past boyfriends. Just general statements when called for—just like he did with his old girlfriends.

The only thing that current Brother Mr. Right will want to hear about your old boyfriend is that he works in the mailroom and has three kids out of wedlock. That will make him happy.

He does not want to know if your ex is a doctor or lawyer or has a television show. Keep it to yourself. Don't give details, don't show pictures, don't even tell names if you can avoid it. Make it so that if you ever passed homeboy on the street, he wouldn't know him from the next stranger walking by.

Besides, you don't want to give your man an up-close-and-personal look at all the baggage you've carried from other relationships, because it'll force him to think that it's something he has to deal with, too. You don't want to send him running, wondering what the hell he got himself into by dating you—

whether you're going to treat him the same way you treated the last guy. You want him to know that history will not repeat itself with him, that you don't intend to hold him accountable for the things that made your last relationship fail. The easiest way to do that is to keep that information to yourself—period.

Now, there are some things he needs to know about if he's going to be in your life—like if you were abused by your last man, or if you were raped. Those are serious issues that have some kind of effect on who you are, and he needs to know these things so that he can be sensitive to your needs, your desires, and what you need to do to continue to heal from those devastating moments in your life. A good man cares about those kinds of things and the well-being of his lady—so tell him.

But everything else? The run-of-the-mill conflicts you had with Robert, or the lack of vacation time with Tyrone? Keep it to yourself.

You'll be thankful you did.

You Don't Wear a Cape, So Don't Try to Be Superwoman

On his seventies album *Inner Visions*, Stevie Wonder had a beautiful mid-tempo ballad called "Superwoman"—about a chick named Mary who, as her dreams were being deferred, pushed her man out of her way so that she could deal with her problems on her own.

She was, after all, Superwoman, and she didn't need any man to deal.

"Very well," Stevie sang with that sweet tenor.

By the end of the song, she finally hears what he's saying and claims she's changed—but he dumps her anyway because he knows that "tomorrow will reflect love's past." He sings his good-bye and he's out.

Twenty years ago, Stevie used his song to tap into a few raw nerves and give voice to brothers fed up with Superwoman sistahs who put on their capes and fly straight through life's adversities—ignoring the fact that their men want to play an active role in keeping them from crashing and burning. Perhaps Stevie should re-release his song.

More than ever, sistahs are bringing home their own bacon, frying it in the pans they purchased with their own money, and going out of their way to forget that he's a man. They don't need him for anything—because they can get what they want on their own, thank you very much. If he can hang, fine; if he can't, screw him because life will go on with or without him.

We get this, in part, from our mothers. They, after all, are the ones who taught us sistahs to be fiercely independent—to expect nothing of anyone else, especially black men. All our lives, we've been told by our mamas—and shown by all too many of our fathers—that we have to go it alone, that if we want to succeed and acquire the finer things in life, we have to get them for ourselves because no black man is capable of getting them for us. We've been disappointed so often by the absence of our fathers and the absence of emotional support from men that we've grown up promising ourselves that we will never again place ourselves in a position of needing or relying on a man.

So we put up layers of protection. We keep our men from getting inside. It's a natural instinct to just go on ahead and get what we want for ourselves, without having to depend on some man to screw up the game plan.

Meanwhile, while Mommy was raising us, she was loving our brothers, teaching them that it was okay to both need women and be needed by them, to be a man.

And the signals, obviously, get crossed.

So we get up early, fix the kids breakfast, get them off the school, go to the job, let the boss work our nerves to the point where we want to kill him, come home, cook, clean, get the kids ready for bed, then catch our breath long enough to sit back for two minutes and brood silently about how jacked up our day was. Then we pick ourselves up and start all over again, no matter how much we just want to sit back down.

And we do it alone, whether we have a man or not. Our capes enable us to do so.

Well, aren't there some days, sistah, when you want to just sit back, rest your head on his shoulder, and at least let him know what you've gone through? To be able to take that cape off, let your guard down, and cry or scream or even laugh about it with someone? You have no problem doing it with the girls. How about trying it with your man?

That is, after all, one of the reasons you have a man in the first place. He's supposed to be in your corner, to listen to you—be attentive to your needs, your ambitions, your desires—and to help you reach those goals. Not taking advantage of that would be like spending forty thousand dollars on a beautiful Land Rover, then leaving it parked in the garage while you drive the beat-up, ten-year-old Hyundai.

Why waste all that money and energy on a new car you're never going to use?

If you don't break the cycle and allow yourself to trust a man and need him, you may very well chase him away, because every man needs to feel needed—particularly black men, who are constantly told by society that they are unimportant, unnecessary (unless they can shoot a basketball), and irrelevant. The last thing he needs is to come home and be treated the same way by his lady.

Now, I'm not suggesting you run screaming and crying to your man every time something goes wrong; nobody likes a neurotic person. And I also have to make it clear that it's okay for Sistahs' Rules girls to be strong black women. We've carried immeasurable weight on our backs from the slave ships, the cotton fields, and the sit-ins to our careers on Wall Street and our space on the welfare line, and that's not going to change anytime soon.

But every now and then, sistahs, it's okay to take off the cape and let your man know that you do need him there, that he's welcome to be in your corner—that he is as invaluable to you as you are to him.

That cape, after all, won't be able to keep you warm 24-7-365.

Never Ask a Question You Don't Want the Answer To

A quiz:

   Scenario No. 1 It's a cool Thursday evening. You and your Brother Mr. Right have just finished a fabulous dinner over at his place and you two are sipping wine as you reminisce about the wild and crazy days of your misspent youth. He pulls out his collection of old photos to show you those scandalous family reunion pictures—the ones with him in the jherri curl, sucking on a rib, cheesing with his crazy Uncle Pookie. Like a sign from God, a picture of some babe with a smile that's slightly bigger than the skimpy, micro-mini bikini she's donning on some exotic beach falls out of the pile. On the back, it says "Bermuda, 1991 . . . Love Jennifer."

Do you:

A) Ask who the hell Jennifer is and if he's talked to her since you two have been dating.

B) Leave it the hell alone.

Scenario No. 2 It's been a really tough month at work, and everybody's been staying late to finish up that big order that's due for shipment like yesterday. Of course, since you've been putting in fifteen-hour days, you haven't had time to hit the gym like you usually do, and you haven't had time to whip up those balanced low-fat meals that, up until now, you've been conscientiously eating. Instead, your fingers are sore from dialing up takeout at that slamming soul food restaurant down the street from the office; your lips have seen more than a little bit of time wrapped around forkfuls of that macaroni and cheese and fattening barbecue chicken and rib platter—and it's starting to show. You've already pushed your favorite jeans to the back of the closet, for you can no longer fit your left leg in them—and the suit you're wearing at this very moment is clinging to your hips like Saran Wrap on a turkey leg.

Do you:

A) Ask your man if he thinks you could stand to lose a coupla pounds.

B) Hit the gym and leave it the hell alone.

Scenario No. 3 You're on the couch wrapped in your baby's arms, a bowl of popcorn in one hand, a pint of Häagen-Dazs in the other. You're comfortable around him, so you don't think twice about flopping into his lap with your hair in a sloppy ponytail, those holey sweatpants and that oversized old-ass New Edition T-shirt you bought the last time they performed in your hometown—about twelve years ago. He flips to BET just in time to catch the height of that new Toni Braxton video—the one where girlfriend has her finely tuned body squeezed into that shiny vinyl body suit, and she's twisting what her mama gave her all up in the camera. Your boyfriend damn near knocks you over trying to lean into the television.

Do you:

A) Ask him if he thinks you're as pretty as Toni.

B) Leave it the hell alone.

Scenario No. 4 You've just moved in with your new fiancé and you two are helping each other unpack your boxes. You come across the box where he holds his old mementos—and immediately tear into it like you don't know what it is. After going through his love letters, you come across a steamy porn tape with an inscription on it from some woman—a suggestive message that clearly indicates homegirl was a freak mama who, at some point, turned your man out.

Do you:

A) Ask him if you're as good in bed as she was.

B) Close the box and leave it the hell alone.

Scenario No. 5 You and your man got into a nasty tiff and broke up. After three months, you both realize you love each other and can't stand to be apart and you happily reconcile. Just as you are telling your girls that you and he are back on, one of them blurts out that your Brother Mr. Right was seen about town with some babe—at the movies, at the restaurant, at the club, at that party you didn't get invited to. You raise an eyebrow, and get real quiet.

Do you:

A) Run to a phone and ask him if he slept with the little hussy.

B) Recognize that you two weren't together and leave it the hell alone.

If you answered "A" to any or all of those questions, girl— you're obviously a glutton for punishment. The only reason you would think to ask for detail about anything from your man's past is if you really, really want your feelings to get hurt. Either that, or you're looking for some kind of guarantee that you are the one and only one he wants. The problem with that is that relationships never come with guarantees. Good ones do come with trust, though. And you don't go around asking stupid questions that could needlessly shatter the trust you two have built.

I mean, come on; you need to know about his past girl-friends and the three-month chippy like Michael Jordan needs a second job. And if you know you need to hit the gym, why ask for his affirmation when you know if he says, "No, honey, you're not gaining weight," you're going to say he's lying, and if he says, "Yes, honey—you do look like you put on a few pounds," you're going to be ticked that he called you fat?

Let's not even get on the Toni Braxton thing.

None of these questions deserve answers because they're none of your business, quite frankly. What he's done in the past was done before he met you—and no matter how scandalous it looks or how pretty she is or what role he played in all of it, the fact of the matter is that as long as he's not doing it while he's with you, you have nothing to say about it. We all have bones in our closet, and we all try really hard to make sure none of them fall out when the person we really care about is sniffing around the door. When one of them accidentally drops on the floor, you, as a responsible, mature, and understanding mate, are supposed to pick it up gingerly and hand it back to him—no questions asked.

Besides, asking him crazy and deranged questions like "Do you think I'm getting fat?" pushes him right into a corner—one in which he will be put into a position of either lying to make you feel better, or telling you the truth and getting you so upset that you wish he lied. What's the benefit?

There is none.

Either way, you're going to get an answer you're not going to appreciate, and he's going to hear it from you—even if he took special care to protect your feelings. Why put yourself through that when you can just leave it alone? Relationships come with enough tension and disagreement and heartache and pain as it is without you adding to it with a bunch of stupid, irrelevant questions like "Am I as cute as Bermuda girl?"

Now, there are, of course, instances where questions are indeed in order. Like when you find lipstick on his collar, or the fruity fragrance on his suit jacket isn't yours. Or when he walks into the house at 2:00 A.M. and that phone number marked Tyra on that book of matches falls out of his pocket. Particularly if her digits keep showing up on your phone bill.

Now that's some red flag stuff to ask about.

That other mess? High school crap.

After all, chances are the closest he'll ever get to Toni is the television screen or the concert-hall seat anyway. Besides, if you're working Rule #3—Hook It Up, Girl!—neither she nor the hotty in the skimpy micro-mini have anything on you anyway.

Channel the Bitch Sessions, Keep a Man

You missed your train because your boss, who pissed you off to the highest of pisstivity today, made you stay late to correct a mistake *he* made. You've walked eight blocks trying to catch a cab, but none of them will pick up your black behind. In the course of those eight blocks, ten brothers with absolutely no respect, no couth, and nothing else better to do with their time got in your face talking about "Hey baby, what's yo name, what's yo sign?" and then called you a bitch when you refused to give up the information and the digits and ignored their asses. The one cab that did decide to give you a ride gave you a hard time because he didn't want to drive to your 'hood, then cursed you out because you didn't give him what he considered a proper tip. You walk into your apartment, and your man is on the couch, watching the game. He looks up, says a cheery "Hey babe! How was your day?" then goes right back to the game—like he really didn't expect or want an answer longer than "Great, thanks!"

What do you do?

If you're a sistah, you probably lay his ass out, let him have a piece of your mind.

You look around the house and ask him why he didn't wash the dishes after he tore up your kitchen fixing himself dinner. You consider this the perfect opportunity to curse him out for leaving his wet towel and his nasty gym socks on the floor after he played tennis with the guys last week. You give him the ole one-two for showing up late for that concert you went to last month.

He has just become the target of your bitch session.

You know that's wrong.

Yes, the world serves up some harsh lessons to sistahs; we go day to day fighting for the respect that is due us for the hard work and sacrifices we make on the job, and for our men, our families, and our friends. We slave in everyplace from the boardrooms to the janitorial closets, on the bank line to the check-cashing line, only to get back to the office, or on the train, or in the street to be treated as if we haven't made some kind of contribution to society today—that we are really nothing in the scheme of things.

And it's trying—particularly when we can't tell the people

putting us through all those changes that they're wrecking our flow.

But that's no excuse for you to channel your bitching at the first person who comes in your face and can take it: your man. He didn't have anything to do with your bad day. His leaving the wet towel on the bed didn't have anything to do with your boss questioning your abilities. His showing up late to the theater last month had nothing to do with those idiots out on the corner calling you a bitch. His leaving the dirty dishes spread across the kitchen wouldn't have made any of the cab drivers that passed you by be more likely to stop.

He had nothing to do with all the bad things that happened to you in the course of the day, and transferring your hostility and anger to him isn't going to make you or him feel any better. In fact, he'll just become one more person to be mad at. And he—well, you'll have successfully provoked him into shooting from the hip right back at you: He'll respond with bewilderment—"What the hell did I do?"—and react with anger by reminding you of a few thoughtless things you've done over the past few weeks—things he wasn't even thinking about until you jumped bad on him.

The words will be ugly. You'll both say things you'll regret. And the next thing you know, you'll be in a standoff that may take you two weeks to forever to recover from.

All because the boss, the guys on the corner, and the taxicab drivers pissed you off and you decided to take it out on him.

What you need to learn is how to channel the anger at the

person who made you angry—rather than your man. If the boss has made you angry or put unreasonable pressure on you, tell him about it (but in a way that won't get you fired). If the guys on the corner are harassing you, cross the street and ignore them. If the cab driver passes you by or gives you a hard time, take down his license plate number and report his butt to his superiors.

Then come home, tell your baby you need to get some things that happened to you at work off your chest, and let him be your sounding board—the one who provides the sympathetic ear when you're upset, the one who provides the shoulder for you to lean on when it gets kind of thick, the one who helps you find solutions to those things that drive you absolutely batty. Now I'm not saying that you can't let a man know what's on your mind when he's done something wrong. Quite the contrary. If he's messing up, set him straight. If he's consistently late, or he leaves his clothes lying around the house and doesn't clean up after himself, or he doesn't do what he says he's going to do when you need him to do it—let him know. But there's no need to be overly critical, screaming and shouting and carrying on to get your point across. It just takes up too much time and energy that could be better spent making yourself and your man happy.

Above all else, remember this: A Sistahs' Rules girl recognizes that she can't be Superwoman all the time—that looking to her man for advice and support is a source of stability, not a sign of weakness.

Victoria learned the hard way. She'd been having problems on the job for months; she wanted to move to a different department because she felt her current boss was underutilizing her skills and holding her back from lucrative promotions—but he did everything within his power to undercut her and thwart her move. She became increasingly frustrated by it but never confronted her boss out of fear that she would lose her job. So she took to volunteering to do work for the other department on her down time, so that she could prove that she was capable of handling that office's demanding and rigorous schedule.

One night, after staying until almost midnight to finish up her work, Victoria walked outside her job and tried to hail a cab—but none would stop. After she had stood outside in the cold for a half hour, one finally did stop, but the driver tried to kick her out of the cab when he found out she was going into Brooklyn. She talked him into going, but he fought her all the way—putting the already tired and upset Victoria over the edge. By the time the cab arrived at Victoria's house, she was threatening to get her boyfriend to come out and beat up the cab driver because he had called her a bitch. But when she called Rich out, he obviously hadn't any clue as to how bad Victoria's day had been or that she'd had a blowup argument with the driver. She told Rich to kick the cab driver's ass; he paid the guy and told him to leave.

Needless to say, that's all Victoria needed to tell Rich off. She was angry at him for not hitting the guy, angry at him for letting the man get away with calling her a bitch, angry at him for not supporting her—so she went into the apartment, snatched a comforter out of the closet, and slept on the sofa. For the third time that month, Victoria was accusing Rich of not supporting her—even though the root of her anger was her boss, her job, and the exhaustion she was suffering from being overworked. The cab driver was the catalyst, but Rich was the fall guy.

Rich was obviously undone. In five minutes, he had gone from sitting up after hours waiting patiently to greet his baby after a hard day's work to sleeping in a cold bed—alone. He just couldn't take it anymore.

The next morning when Victoria woke up, she was greeted with a long letter from Rich saying he was tired of being her whipping boy when things went wrong on the job.

"I'll arrange to pick up my things later this weekend," the letter ended.

Victoria never did get that new job; she quit before she could get transferred. My friend Rich is now with a woman who respects him enough to listen to his advice and is strong enough to ask for his shoulder when things aren't working well. He does the same for her.

They've built a terrific relationship—one that Victoria dreams about every night while she's home alone, complaining about how she can't find a good man.

Her bed is going to stay cold.

Don't let yours end up that way too.

Be His Lover, Not His Mother

He's endured years of being nagged to clean his room, wash the dishes, pick up his clothes, and pick his friends with care. Today, when he comes home to his own apartment, he's not expecting that nagging to continue in his own abode—particularly if it's coming from his woman.

So don't do it.

He moved away from home because he grew up; he can make his own decisions, work at his own pace—clean when he wants to and leave the dirty dishes in the sink until he gets good and ready to wash them. The only woman on earth who is allowed to tell him what to do is his

mother—and as an adult, he listens to her maybe only half the time.

If the brother isn't going to listen to his mama, what makes you think he's going to listen to your whining and nagging?

See, a brother likes to feel he has some sort of control over his career, over his household, over his choice in friends—and if you start questioning his decisions and telling him what to do, he'll start doubting himself or, worse yet, stop taking anything you have to say seriously. That could lead him to make a few stinging decisions of his own—namely, stop asking your opinion, stop sharing his feelings and news with you, and ultimately, resent you.

What kind of relationship would that be if you couldn't be there for him? You already know that Rule #23—Be His Homie—is of the utmost importance—that his ability to depend and lean on you when it gets thick is central to the relationship. He needs you to listen, be attentive, and offer that shoulder—without ramming your self-righteous opinions down his throat. What you have to do is let him fly his own plane, make his own decisions and live by his own rules—within reason, of course—or make it so that you two devise your rules together and live by them accordingly, without nagging each other to follow them to a T.

So that you'll know when you're being helpful and when you need to just shut the hell up, I've devised a four-step plan for "Knowing When You've Crossed the Mama-Knows-Best

Line." It'll help you figure out when you're acting like his girl-friend/lover/fiancée/wife, and when you're acting like his mama.

You're Babying Him

Say he lost his job, or he didn't get that promotion he was counting on. He comes home, bottom lip poked out, in a funky mood and not really wanting to talk about it. Finally, he sits down on the couch, and in between sipping his beer and flipping through the television channels, he says it: "I didn't get the job." Don't keep quiet and walk out the room; that's unfeeling. He told you for a reason. But whatever you do, don't plop down on the couch and stroke his head and coo and tell him, "It's going to be all right, baby—those fools don't know they're missing out on the best thing that ever could have happened to the company if they'd picked you." That's something his mother would say—and now is not the time for stroking him and making him feel like an even bigger failure than he's already pegged himself to be. Do tell him that there's always another job, or another promotion, and that you have every confidence in the world that he's smart enough and strong enough to find something even better—then leave it at that. You'll have boosted his ego and given him room to either talk about it some more or drop it on his own—without getting him more worked up by offering to go blow up his boss's house. Nothing good ever comes out of that—but letting him deal with it on his own, while, in the back of his mind, he knows you're there for him if he needs it, well, that feels pretty good to a brother.

You're Ordering Him to Do Something and Telling Him How to Do It

I had a friend who used to put her boyfriend through all kinds of changes with unreasonable demands and expectations. I mean, the boy didn't mind doing for her—but sistah-girl just took it to all kinds of new levels. If she was at her mother's house and the stove needed fixing, she was on the phone, demanding that her man come over and fix it. If her car needed servicing, oh, she wouldn't take it down to the shop; she would call him over and make him do it. If she thought her daughter's room needed a new coat of paint and a nice trim to go around the ceiling's borders? You know he was told to be at her house, paintbrush in hand. And even though she knew nothing about stoves, cars, and painting, she always took it on herself to stand over brother's shoulder and tell him what to do. "Why are you pulling the stove out?" she'd ask. "Why'd you take it to that shop? You could have saved two dollars if you'd driven to the next town over," she'd criticize. "That's the wrong color—I said egg white, not eggshell," she'd say as she rolled her eyes and folded her arms. She had old boy so turned around after a while, he didn't know what to do. I mean, his own mama didn't order him around like that—and his mom was pretty damn bossy. One day, brother just started finding reasons for why he couldn't come around—why he couldn't carry her laundry down to the basement, why he couldn't take her grocery shopping, why he couldn't baby-sit her kid while she went shopping. He didn't need that mess; he'd finished playing Cinderella the day he moved out of his bossy mama's house—and he wasn't about to get into a serious relationship with a woman who bossed him just as much as she did. Moral of the story: Don't treat your man like he's Cinderella; share the household responsibilities and, if you can't do it and you somehow manage to talk him into doing it, at least act like you appreciate it.

Don't Be Overly Critical

I know a guy who would do anything for his baby—anything. Still, his girlfriend never thought it was enough. She would find fault with everything he did for her and frequently accuse him of not caring enough about her because he didn't jump as soon as she hinted she wanted him to do her a favor. Finally, she pushed him over the edge. Her car was clearly on its last legs—or at least one of its major parts made it seem like it was. After starting it and hearing the car make a noise that sounded like a really sick mule, she came into the house and told her man she was taking the car to the shop because something was obviously wrong with it. She really wanted him to offer to take it for her—but she gave no indication that was her intention. So she huffed out of the house, took the car to the shop herself, then came back and reamed old boy out for not being supportive enough. The world didn't end, the car was fixed, and she didn't lose any time fretting over it—yet she was hell-bent on criticizing him for not doing something he had no idea he was supposed to do. This was nothing new to him, though; she was famous for desiring something from him but not asking him to do it, then accusing him of not caring for her when he didn't automatically jump to perform whatever duties she was looking for him to perform. But on this day, he just got tired of getting reamed out for not being one of those mind readers on the psychic hot line. So he stepped. The point here is that you can't constantly criticize someone for not caring for you or not doing what you think he's automatically supposed to do, and expect him not to feel like he's being nagged. I'm not saying don't express your feelings; if you need to tell him about himself, then do it. But don't do it in that nasal, nagging, "You don't love me because you woulda, coulda, shoulda" kinda way, because that's the way of mothers. Save it for your kids.

Never Love a Man Unconditionally

Mothers love their crackhead kids. Mothers love their jailbird sons. Mothers love their alcoholic, abusive, no-good offspring.

They have to; it's their nature. No mother is going to turn her back on the child she carried for nine months and raised for upwards of eighteen years.

You don't have to do that.

If he's abusive, if he's addicted to drugs or alcohol, if he's no good—it is not your job to love him unconditionally. It is your job to demand that he either get help or step, because you don't need that in your life. A mother can never replace her son; you can replace a man. Just do it.

Four simple rules, guaranteed to keep you out of the "Mom Zone." Remember them, use them; they'll save him a whole lot of grief—and ultimately, you too.

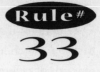
Rule # 33

Getting to Know His Mother and Sisters Goes a Long Way

We knew it wasn't right, but we did it anyway. We couldn't help it.

My mom and I loved my brother Troy's now-ex-girlfriend, and we did everything within our power to try to keep them together. Mommy liked her because she was sweet and caring, smart and willing to please my brother—all the things a mother ever wished for her son. I liked her because she was young like me, had energy, and knew better than to take any of his mess.

So when things didn't go right between them, we had her back—or, at the very least, gave her the benefit of the doubt.

Hey, my mom and I adore Troy—but we loved

her, too. And let me tell you, it did wonders for her when something stupid went down in their relationship and she needed that extra nudge to help him get over whatever it was he needed to get over.

Likewise, we shunned the dating and outright mentioning of any hootchie other than the woman we considered Troy's "The One." If he brought someone other than "The One" to the house, we made a point of treating her, well, like she wasn't "The One."

That's, of course, what you want—a sister and mother who are on your side, who like you, who have your back. They're your first and last line of defense—the ones who, if you play your cards right, do all the blocking for your relationship. Again, what you have to recognize and remember is that brothers, more likely than not, have very special relationships with their mothers—and, in some cases, their sisters. These are the first two females they'll have had sustained contact with. His mother, hopefully, will have taught him how to treat women and, by setting herself up as an example of a good black woman, how to spot a good one for himself. His sister, through her relationships with other guys, will have taught him the ways of young women—how they react to the everyday trials and tribulations of young black couples falling in and out of love, how they look first thing in the morning. He may seek her out for advice, or he may scope out her interactions with guys from afar—but, in some way or another, he will get some useful hints from her on how to handle women.

And when he brings you home to meet his two favorite girls, it's sort of his final test—the one that tells him if you're truly the one he should keep around. You know you're there for a reason; no man is going to put himself and another human being through the agonizing family gamut of scrutiny unless he's really, really considering staying in this relationship for the long haul. If, at the end of the family meeting, Mom and Sis whisper sweetly in his ear that they like you, oh—you're in there.

My mother-in-law, Migozo, tells me that she was genuinely in love with her then-boyfriend, Chikuyu, a jazz musician whom she'd met in Boston, when he announced that he wanted to take her to meet his mother, Mary. Migozo says she was scared as heck—and she had a long train ride all the way to Jersey City, New Jersey, to think about what she was going to say and how she was going to act in front of the mother of the man she loved.

When they finally arrived, Migozo walked in and shyly introduced herself, and said something like "pleased to meet you." They exchanged pleasantries and had a perfectly lovely afternoon. Days later, one of Chikuyu's sisters would tell her brother, "You better marry that girl." It didn't take too much longer before he did.

Moral of the story: First impressions are everything.

Imagine if Mama Mary had said she didn't like Migozo. Suppose the sister didn't like her, either. Not to say that Chikuyu wouldn't have married her, but it certainly would have made him think twice about the woman he was planning on spending the rest of his life with. And certainly if he'd gone through with it without his mother's nod, it could have gotten pretty funky. In his quest to keep everyone happy, he'd have made sure that Migozo and Mary had as little contact as possible. No visits. Few phone calls. And Mary, like any other mother with sense, would have figured that no-good woman took her son away from her, and would have disliked her even more.

Snowball effect.

Folks in situations like that don't know what to do once they're in it. When they get around each other at family gatherings, everyone's hypersensitive to what the other says, and folks tend to take little things out of context—in a big way.

The girlfriend thinks the mother and sister are being stank. The mother and sister think likewise. Brotherman is caught all up in the middle—uncomfortable as all get out.

And it gets worse when there're kids around—as Grandma and Auntie will swear that no-good woman of his is keeping them away from their flesh and blood. The implications are far-reaching.

Avoid it.

When you get there, know how to act. Sucking up isn't bad. But a more realistic approach would be to simply be yourself and, above all else, treat his mama and sister like you'd like him to treat yours. Be polite, be gracious—and for goodness' sake, act like you've got some home training. You don't want to give Mom and Sis any excuse to talk about your butt. Make conversation. Feel them out: If Mom is a talker and likes to discuss today's current events, keep up with her. If she's not the talkative type, speak to her—but don't overdo it. If she offers you the chance to do intimate things with her—like baste the turkey before she sets the Thanksgiving dinner, or go shopping for a few groceries—do it.

It certainly won't hurt your case any.

I'd like to believe that I didn't suck up any when I first met my man's parents—but I do remember being nervous and secretly praying that they'd like me. I tried to strike that perfect balance—to be talkative but not a jabberjaw, sweet but not syrupy, funny but not goofy. We ended up having a ball. During my first visit, his younger sister was getting married—so it was really easy for me to fit in during such a joyous occasion.

Luckily, his mother was a sweet, down-to-earth woman, and his sisters were really cool. We hit it off lovely. And when his father dropped us off at the airport after our visit, he whispered in my ear during our warm good-bye embrace that the family "loves you."

It brought tears to my eyes, because it was important for me to know that they love me just as much as I love them.

Shack Up

So you think you know him, huh?

Try living with his butt.

See, that other stuff—that commitment and honesty and trust—is cute when you two aren't in each other's face 24-7. You go on your dates, take your trips, and sleep at each other's houses, and everything is just dandy. You have a drawer for your underwear at his spot, and he has a space carved out in your closet for his shirts and slacks—and you're both really good at picking your things up and folding and hanging them neatly. You go to sleep in your cute little teddies, your hair slightly askew but still nice—then wake up before he does so that you can brush those teeth, clean out those eye boogers, and wash that face before he can get a good glimpse of your morning mug, pre–makeup brush. And if you're in a funky mood, you stay at your own crib and set a date for when you're feeling a bit better about life, yourself, and him—then continue the relationship as if it's the greatest union since Heathcliff and Clair on *The Cosby Show*.

Basically, you and he are stepping lightly. Both of you do everything you can to make the other think that this relationship is workable—that you two are really good for one another. You both hide that other stuff—sloppiness, attitude, emotional baggage, responsibility, neurosis, your therapists' names—and you put on those rose-colored glasses and your best foot forward so that you can get down to the business of loving your mate.

All that superficial, fake stuff disappears real quick, though, when you move in with him. You just can't keep all that crap—the niceness, the neatness, the rosy, picture-perfect relationship—going all the time when you live with someone. Eventually and inevitably, you're both going to have to lay the cuteness to the side and let the other person see you—all of you. When that happens, you get a pretty good indication of whether your mate is really the person you want to spend the rest of your life with, or if you want to kill him and assume another identity in another state.

Now, if your mama and you are anywhere as old-fashioned as my mama, you're not going to go for living with a man to whom you're not married. The motto you'll hurl at him and anyone else who will listen is an oldie but goodie: "Why buy the cow if you can get the milk for free?"

The answer is that you want to make sure the milk isn't spoiled.

You want to know his quirks, his likes, his dislikes, his rituals and his habits—the good ones and the bad ones. You want to know if he's responsible, you want to know if he handles his money properly or if he's going to run your good credit into the ground. You want to know if he's truly true to this relationship and willing to work through the good times as well as the really ugly ones—and how he's going to deal with all your stank rituals, habits, attitudes, and faults.

You'll never truly understand and appreciate any of that if you continue to pay separate rents.

Shortly after they got engaged, Angelou and James moved in with one another. They were law students at the University of Florida College of Law and decided that since they were together all the time anyway, they should shack up to save on rent. In hindsight, though, both of them readily admit that their moving in together was about much more than the combining of leases; this was their trial—a mini-marriage of sorts—that was going to help verify that they truly wanted to spend the rest of their lives with each other.

She was more carefree about hanging out with the girls; he wanted to know where she was all the time. He didn't like that she wasn't as neat as he; she didn't like that he was such a neat freak. And on top of all that, they were trying to get through law school—arguably one of the most difficult tasks either of them ever took on, ever.

Their union remained intact. After they took the masks off and exposed their hearts for one another to see, they figured out in that year they lived together that, in the scheme of things, their love for and desire to be with one another far outweighed that other mess. And they both say they're glad they took that chance.

Of course, it takes a lot of serious labor to make living together work. It's like having a roommate, but way more intense because you two actually spend the majority of your time together. You can't go into your room and he into his, close the door and not be seen by the other for days at a time—because you are, for all intents and purposes, husband and wife without the license, ceremony, and rings. You sleep in the same bed, you eat at the same time, you socialize together—you plan and do everything for two. You can't ignore one another, you can't stay mad at one another, you can't kill one another, because the challenge here is to make it work. When you're dating someone and there's no investment in the relationship, he is dismissible. But if you're living with him, well, you're more apt to work it out because you feel compelled to and so does he. You've both invested a lot of time, energy, and money into this relationship—and neither of you is going to feel comfortable just jumping up, packing your stuff, calling the moving company, finding another apartment, forgetting about each other, and starting another relationship without first making the effort to fix what's wrong.

Sometimes, of course, it doesn't work out—no matter how hard you try.

Take, for instance, Nicole and Dean. Everything was hunky-dory between the two when they were dating. They also went to school together—Yale—and after they graduated, they decided to stay together and see if they could build toward marriage. They moved in together a year out of college—and on the surface, everything appeared to be just fine. But then, her career started faltering; she couldn't find a comfortable place in the workforce and she was starting to feel like she was working hard but getting nowhere fast.

Dean ended up being the target of her frustration, and neither his skin nor his stomach was thick or strong enough to sustain her emotional wrath. She turned out to be an evil, nasty somebody who made both of them miserable. They ended up hating each other but holding on for the sake of holding on— until they just couldn't hold on anymore.

The good thing here is that they realized it and went their separate ways. The only thing they had to break was a lease. Imagine if they didn't recognize the problems until after they were married. It would have been another black marriage down the drain—and the only way they could have walked away from each other was through the courts. So in Nicole and Dean's case, living together was actually a good tool in determining that they weren't put on this earth for each other.

God did put me on this earth for my honey, though. We'd dated for slightly less than a year when we decided that it was too stupid for us to continue maintaining two apartments when we were, most of the time, using only one. If I wasn't at his house, he was at mine. It only made sense that we move in together.

Of course, I have my faults and he has his—but nothing so serious that we'd want to fire one another. What our living together did was bring us even closer together—make us realize that this was a good, strong, healthy relationship that just got better with time. Our friendship grew, our bond grew—our love grew—and we found that we were just so much more happy with each other than we were without each other.

He proposed just a few months into our second lease.

I'm no fool.

Share the Household Responsibilities

Depending on a man to pay all the bills in your house is played out like the eight-track.

Ditto for you being responsible for all the cooking and cleaning in the house, and the day-to-day rearing of the children.

This is the nineties, for God's sake—you're not his maid, he's not your personal bank account. This is the challenge of our era: Both of you are not only capable of—but are—bringing home the bacon and frying those suckers up in the pan. Both of you have to recognize and respect the newfangled roles that we've taken on as double breadwinners in a world fraught with big expenses, little time, and a serious need for shared responsibility.

When we were little, it was a lot more clear-cut: Our fathers worked, came home, ate our mothers' food, played with us, relaxed with a few cold ones, then went to bed. Our mothers, most of whom were forced to work to help keep the family's financial ship afloat, came home from a hard day's work to a second job—one where they were required to cook, feed the kids and help them with their homework, get them ready for bed, bust suds in the kitchen, tidy up the house, and then, and only then, hit the sack. On the weekends, he would mow the lawn; and she would clean the house from top to bottom, hit the grocery store, and assume her role as chief Lord of the Kids.

Everybody knew—and had—their place.

Well, those days are O.V.E.R. Over.

Dead and stinkin'.

Outta here.

Today, you, my dear sistah, may be drawing a bigger salary than his and spending more time at work than he does, too. When you come home from work, you just may want him to have dinner and a cold one waiting for you.

And there's nothing wrong with that. Hell, if you've got a good brother at home, he won't mind breaking down and doing that for you, either.

But this isn't a perfect world, and fantasy almost always takes a backseat to reality. So in the real world, I suggest you lay down some real ground rules.

The key word here, sistahs?

Share.

In a relationship, democracy is a beautiful thing—and it's up to you to sit down with your man and set some guidelines on how the politics of housecleaning, cooking, entertaining, and bill paying are going to be handled between you, *before* things get thick.

For instance, if you don't like scrubbing toilets, washing dishes, doing laundry, and all those other nasty, time-consuming chores, and he doesn't either—take turns. Set up a realistic schedule that you both have to follow to a T—like, you take turns washing the dishes every other night, or you clean the bathroom on every first and third Saturday, and he takes the responsibility on every second and fourth Saturday. You pay for the groceries one week, he pays the next. The last person out of the bed in the morning makes the bed. You both go and do the laundry, suffer over the washing machine and dryer together. You cook together, take turns over the hot stove every night, or eat out.

It's that simple.

What's even better is if you can afford to pay someone to do it for you. For instance, when my honey and I moved in together, we set up those schedules but were pretty bad at keeping them. He'd be the one who was supposed to clean the bathroom on Saturday and wouldn't get to it until Tuesday. I'd be the one who was supposed to mop the hardwood floors on Sunday, and I'd find something else to do so that they wouldn't get done until it was his turn to do them. The dishes hardly ever got done until the sink was overflowing—and then the one who got stuck holding the sponge and Palmolive would pitch a bitch between washing and drying.

It got borderline ugly—and had the potential to get much worse, until we did something about it. We agreed to hire a maid to come in and do for us once a week what we hated to do ourselves. We take turns paying her seventy dollars a week to clean our apartment top to bottom, a little extra if we want her to do laundry. The best investment of one hundred and forty dollars a month I could ever think of, because it completely eliminated the tension caused by dirty toilets, sinks full of dishes, and unmopped floors. I've spent that much money on much worse things, trust me. If that's all it takes to keep me and my man from duking it out over chores, so be it.

He cooks, I cook—we both cook when we're hungry, or we eat out. No big deal.

We also agreed up front to share the bills, rather than have one depend on the other to pay them all. It's up to you and your brotherman to decide how you're going to split the finances, but the way we did it was easy: We shared how much our salaries were, then split the rent according to the percentage of money we brought into the house. He took one of the bigger utility bills, and I took all the little ones—which always added up to pretty much the amount of the bill he paid. When we go grocery shopping, we generally split the bill down the middle.

Then I pay my credit card and student loan bills, and he

pays his. We keep separate bank accounts, and he does with his money as he pleases, as I do with mine—until it comes time to pay the bills.

It's that simple.

We haven't had a single fight over money, household chores, or cooking in the years we've been together—and I don't anticipate we will anytime soon. We're too busy enjoying life to be bothered by such minor concerns as these.

If you handle it right, sistah, then you will be able to get your Brother Mr. Right to do the same thing, too.

If he's a good man, he'll appreciate your fairness and your willingness to share in the household's financial responsibilities.

He, in turn, won't have a problem getting with Mr. Clean.

MORE
SISTAHS'
RULES

Leave Her Man Alone

If he has a ring on his finger, ditch him quick.

There is absolutely nothing to be gained for you, sistah, from dating a married man—nothing, that is, except emptiness and heartache.

Think about it: While you're at your parents' house on Christmas, getting grilled by your aunt for not bringing your man over so that the folks can check him out, he's off somewhere with the wife and kids, opening presents and being there for his happy little family.

While he's off for a week down in Virginia at the family reunion with Wifey and Co., you're home wishing it was you that he was introducing to his uncle George and cousin Sophia.

On Valentine's Day, you get flowers sent to your office—from his secretary. She gets the romantic dinner, the wine, and the dessert—at their home.

You see him only when *he* can sneak and see you—and when he does, it's only to have sex, nothing meaningful.

You can't wake up in the morning with him at your side.

You can't go out with him when you want to.

You can't call him when you want to.

You can't depend on him to be there for you.

You can't have him for yourself—and if, by some act of weird, cosmic force you do get him, you can't trust his butt.

All the things that a Sistahs' Rules girl checks off on her wish list when she's searching for her Brother Mr. Right are null and void when it comes to a married man—because the marriage license he signed with his wife makes him somebody else's Brother Mr. Right.

Find your own.

I know that for some sistahs, all of those faults are okay. She likes that the guy isn't in her face all the time, smothering her with affection. She likes the secrecy and excitement of it all—the thrill of doing something that's forbidden. She doesn't mind that he's off with someone else, or several someone elses, when he's not with her.

But you know what? Sistahs' Rules girls don't ever play second fiddle; they're never the side act to the main gig. They know that they are number one, two, three, four, and five in their Brother Mr. Right's life—never runner-up to any other sistah, not even his mama. They know that the man who is lucky enough to have them knows this, too, and will make every effort to deliver.

If he's with her, how on earth would he be able to make you number one in his life? His allegiance will always be with her, she will always come first, because she is the one he said "I do" to, the one who bore his children, the one who's been there for him, the one he loves. Chances are he's not going to leave her if there's nothing drastically wrong with their relationship, and he's just using you to get some on the side.

You can't go out like a sucker believing that he's going to leave her and get with you; he's already proven that he's a liar and can't be trusted. Think about it; while he's out creeping with you, he's probably lied to her about where he is. And Lord knows that if he's out on a date with someone other than his wife and he lied to her about it, he can't be trusted.

Remember: Honesty and trust are at the tippity-top of a Sistahs' Rules girl's wish list.

And say he does end up leaving her and the kids to be with you; what makes you so sure that what you've whipped on him is so good that it will stop him from cheating on you, too? How can you trust that he won't, if you already know for a personal fact that he's capable of doing it and has done it before?

Your Brother Mr. Right is just that: *Your* Brother Mr. Right. He is not to be shared. He is not to disrespect you and your relationship. He is not to make you wonder if, when he calls you from the restaurant, he's really out with Jerome and not Shaniqua. He is not to use you for sex, then shower you with cheap gifts to make up for the fact that he's not there.

He is there for you and only you, and you are there for him and only him.

It's that simple.

If he tells you that he loves you because you listen to and understand him and his wife doesn't, tell him to go see a therapist. If he tells you his wife doesn't treat him right and he needs someone who will, tell him to get a divorce and buy a dog.

You're not in the business of being a substitute. Tell him to get lost, and you go find your own man—someone who will respect you enough to be with you and only you.

I have a girlfriend who was dating a guy who swore up and down he was going to leave his new wife. "I made a mistake and she's just not the right one for me," he told her. "You're my soul mate." He claimed that the reason he married her was because they'd been dating each other since high school, and it was a natural progression in the relationship—but not the right one. My girl believed him, and hung on. He was planning to leave her by Halloween. By October 31, though, wifey was preggers. He was going to talk to her by Thanksgiving and leave her then. By Christmas, he was saying that it was the holiday and he couldn't just drop something like that while they were opening presents. "February, baby—I swear."

Two Februarys, a baby, and another child on the way later, he was still talking about "Next month." And she, like a dummy, continued to wait. She finally left him—but only after another man came into her life and showed her how a lady is supposed to be treated. Boy, that brick fell on her head and she couldn't fire Mr. I'm Leaving, Really fast enough. In hindsight, she realizes how foolish she was—but it's easy to do Monday morning quarterbacking a day after the game is over. What she wished was that she had recognized it sooner, before she wasted two years of her life.

Don't do that to yourself, girl.

He's just not worth it—particularly when the world is full of many more beautiful, trustworthy, attractive, got-it-together men without wives at home.

If He Wants Out or He's Not Acting Right, Show Him the Door

Mary J. Blige put it best when, with that rough, throaty voice of hers, she told her soon-to-be-ex in her smash song "Not Gon' Cry" that she should have "left his ass a thousand times."

Borrowing from the Baptist sistahs who sit up in the front pew early Sunday morning, just calling to pastor, we said, "Weeeell," right on with her.

Girlfriend had us feeling those words—feeling them for all the times we stuck with that trifling, no-good Negro who did us wrong and knew he didn't want to be there, but kept us hanging on anyway. We, like Mary, knew we should have "left his ass a thousand times," but something kept telling us to hang on.

Perhaps it was all those statistics and stories and books and reports telling us that the pool of good black men is so shallow that we have a better chance of being struck by lightning than finding one for ourselves.

Perhaps it's because we sistahs have been conditioned to believe that if we're not in a serious relationship or on our way to being married by a certain age, something is wrong with us.

Perhaps it's because we're afraid of being alone.

Whatever the reason, we hold on to him for dear life—as if his lying, philandering, using, cheating, and general abuse is better than having to go it solo.

Now, don't get me wrong; there's something to be said for working out the kinks in a relationship. Some things, particularly your man, are worth fighting for. I'm not suggesting that when you have an argument with your man, you tell him to get to steppin', and I'm certainly not saying that you shouldn't give him second chances.

But if you've gotten to chance number twenty and he's still not acting right, somebody needs to take some action—and that somebody is you.

Weeeell.

He's seeing other people and you're supposed to be in a committed relationship, you say? He's got to go.

He doesn't go out with you, he's always irritated with you,

and he limits his affection to hittin' it and running? Oh, yeah, he's got to go, girl.

His boys take priority over you, he's immersing himself in work, and you've been with him for years and there's still no ring on that finger?

Need I say it again?

There comes a time when you've got to move on, black girl—move on. Know when to say when, and know when which when is enough. Recognize your limits, and let him know when he's trampled over yours like Evander did Tyson in the third round. Sistahs' Rules girls are never in the business of keeping a man who doesn't want to be kept. If he mistreats you, he doesn't want to be with you, he doesn't want to make it work—or at least he isn't trying his hardest to make it work—well, brother's got to go.

Weeeell.

Don't be afraid, sis. The fear that you'll never find another because there aren't any more brothers out there is misguided. In the now immortal words of the great leader Malcolm X, you've been "hoodwinked, bamboozled—led astray." Don't believe the hype, girl—because they are out there; and in this book, I've given you every secret I know for how to find them, how to meet them, how to get them, and how to keep them.

You're going to have to use those secrets if you want another one—and the sooner you kick Mr. Know No Good to the curb, the sooner you can get to finding your Brother Mr. Right.

Weeeell.

A friend of a friend of mine wasted a good deal of her time and money holding on. She's a twenty-eight-year-old lawyer—a beautiful sistah with her own practice, a line of prestigious clients, and what appears to be an impressive life. But she's convinced herself that she's nothing without a man—that somehow she's not complete unless she has a brother to call her own. Of course, her arduous search for Brother Mr. Right turned into a search for Mr. Anybody Will Do—and she ended up with a real flake who took advantage of her and their relationship and had her so turned out that she didn't know if she was coming or going.

He didn't have a job, but he lied to her and said he did.

Somehow, all of his belongings ended up moved into her spacious apartment, and she was shacking up with a guy that she wasn't too sure she wanted to be shacking up with—but she was happy because he was there.

He took to borrowing money from her account and never returning it, borrowing her car and not coming home at night, or, just as bad, coming home late with Maybelline on his collar, Hennessey on his breath, and CK1 on his jacket—none of which she used.

It was obvious to everyone—including this sistah—that ol' boy was using her, didn't care about her, and had something, perhaps a lot of things, going on on the side. My friend says her friends lent her sympathetic shoulders at first, then quietly started telling her to get rid of him. Finally, they took to just outright dissing him and telling her that she could do better—

way better. But she kept him around because her fear of being an attractive, on-point-but-all-alone sistah just tore her up inside.

What tore her up even more, though, was coming home early from work and catching him—in her bed, mind you—with some other hootchie. After she finished cussing them like she was the devil herself, she sat in her house and cried and cried and cried some more. She knew it was eventually going to come to this—she'd seen all the warning signs, heard all her friends' reservations, known she should have left his ass a thousand times. Still, here she was, her heart torn into itty-bitty pieces.

Don't you know that after a couple of weeks or so, he slithered on back to the house begging her forgiveness? Don't you know she actually considered it?

Weeeell.

Sistahs' Rules girls know better. There's not a man on this earth worth all that heartache.

Even Mary recognized that—told that man that she wasn't "gon' cry, not gon' cry, I'm not gon' shed no tears.

"I can do better," she sang, the pain piercing her word.

So can you, sistah. So can you.

So You Got Dissed, Huh? Get Over It!

You shook him, or perhaps, he beat you to it.

No matter who did what, he's gone—out of your life. And here you stand, alone, heart in hand and no man. What do you do now?

A true Sistahs' Rules girl would use this time to get her constitution together—a personal document that would focus on her plan to repair and reflect on self.

Start with a good cry. That's right—shed some tears. It's okay to cry; it's natural. Any person who tells you that it's a weak response for a weak person is fooling herself. Crying is cleansing; it lets you get out those emotions and that pain, rather than keep them pent up inside. Remember, Sistahs' Rules girls don't wear capes and they're not Superwoman (at least not all the time), and they know that it's perfectly natural to break down every once in a while. If there's ever a time for that, it's now.

But it's not meant to last forever. It's the first step in repairing you. Once you've gotten that out of your system, it's time to get down to the business of taking care of you.

Join a social club. Get a hobby. Hang out with your friends. Read. Shop. Do whatever it is that will relax you—allow yourself time with yourself to improve upon yourself, to get comfortable with being with you—without all the compromises that come with relationships.

Which means, above all else, you avoid jumping into another relationship right away.

No rebounding, under any circumstances whatsoever!

You know those kind of relationships have all the staying power of a Popsicle in the sticky hands of a five-year-old on a hot, southern afternoon. All the baggage that you took from that last relationship will get dumped squarely in his lap. What's he going to do with it—other than throw it back and run like hell? Then you're stuck with another broken heart, and bitterness toward anything with a penis and legs.

My girl Caryl did that. She was engaged to a man for two years—the love of her life, the man whose children she was planning to bear. But, alas, it didn't work out.

Naturally, she was heartbroken when it was over. She had

worn the ring, she had made the plans, and she had even bought the dress—and suddenly, it was over.

But she found another within months—and found herself saying yes to his offering of engagement just a few months after dating him. I don't need to tell you that that one didn't last any longer than the courting stage.

No, rebounding just isn't the move.

Get yourself together mentally. Work on your body. Exude beauty—on the inside and the out—and don't focus on finding another man.

You'll be amazed at how fast this, alone, will bring you another one.

Guys pick up on it when you look hungry—when your eyes are darting everywhere, checking out every guy in the room to see if your husband is anywhere in a ten-feet radius from you. It's funny, but you know how it goes: You're not involved with anyone and you're looking desperate for love and attention—and nary a man pays you any mind. Then the moment you get a man, everyone's trying to throw you phone numbers and time. Brothers do that because they're more attracted to a woman who doesn't make finding a man the focus of her existence. She's perfectly happy with or without a man—and confident that she will eventually get one, without having to put herself out there too far to find him.

That's what you have to do after you've dumped your last one; pick yourself up, dust yourself off, sit down and rest a bit, reflect on the injury, nurse yourself back to health, then go ahead and jump back in when you're sure you're ready.

And when you are, flip on back over to Rule #4, shore up your wish list, and start all over again—confident that you will find someone better than the last, using Sistahs' Rules.

Rules for High School Sistahs

I've got one rule for you: Leave those little boys alone!

Okay, let me stop—I'm trippin'. I know you're not going to listen to that, because you are, after all, high school girls, and that sounds like something your mama would tell you, right?

I know the deal: Boys are your life. Being popular is your life. Being seen hanging on the arm of the most popular guys in the midst of the beautiful people is even more important to you than what's happening on the next episodes of *All My Children*, *Beverly Hills 90210*, *Moesha*, and *Martin* combined.

You want and need to fit in, and he's the one who's going to get you there.

Understood. I was the same way. And I wished to goodness someone would lay out some rules for me so that I could snatch up the attention of Sean Jordan, whom I fell madly in love with from the moment I walked into Oak Park Elementary School in the fifth grade.

Oh, he was beautiful; he had this chocolate-brown skin and these beautiful doe eyes. He was tall (enough) and dressed really cool. And any girl—whether she be black, white, Latino, or otherwise—who dated him was indeed recognized as "the woman" for the length of the relationship.

Alas, ol' boy never paid me any kind of mind.

In fact, I was somewhat of a geek—at least borderline geek. I was smart. I wasn't all that cute (although my mother insists that I was—but she's supposed to say that), I was shy when it came to guys, and everyone was scared to death of my big brother, Troy, who was extremely handsome, extremely popular, and extremely big enough to kick the butt of any guy who mistreated his lil' sis. Basically, I was doomed from day one.

You don't have to be. Here are the Top 10 do's and don'ts for you to keep in mind as you make your way through the high school fire:

1. Study and get good grades. Even though I thought it was a major stumbling block in the middle of my road when I was in high school, I'm still convinced that that was the best thing I ever did. The guys who are worth it are going to appreciate a smart young lady—and if they don't, well, hey—you'll go off to college and come back with a degree and the beginnings of a good career, and he'll be still sitting in the same spot with the same tired, stupid girl who didn't have sense enough but to follow behind a dummy.

2. Get involved with extracurricular activities and sports. It's a great way to meet guys who like what you like—and it looks good on the college application. Also, go to parties, hit up the basketball and football games, participate in all the social events that will put you in the circles with other students—they get to know you that way, and you get to be seen.

3. Stay fit, be healthy. You can't front; guys love a sistah with a nice body and clear skin and natural beauty. Why deny them—and particularly yourself—any of that? Exercise and eat those chitterlings and fried pork chops in moderation, because more than a few moments with those on your lips will put a lifetime of weight on those hips and pimples on that face if you don't watch it. Keep your hair and nails done; take care of you. When you take care of you, he'll notice it. Trust me.

4. Dress hip, but create your own style. It's okay to dress like the beautiful people in those magazines, but if you take it a step further and create your own look, you'll be amazed at how quickly people will copy your style—an automatic popularity draw.

5. Keep 'em closed. Having sex with him will not make him like you any more or any less. High school boys just go with whoever will give it up—and you don't want that kind of reputation because guys will date you simply because you're easy, not because they really like you. I don't need to tell you that's not a boyfriend.

6. *If you are having sex, protect yourself.* If I had my way, this wouldn't even be an issue because none of you would be having sex. But you are. What you need to recognize is that you are among one of the fastest-growing groups of people with AIDS: black children and teenagers. You're also the ones who have a disproportionately high number of out-of-wedlock births. You don't want to get sick, and I know you don't want to be taking care of any babies when you could be out enjoying life and growing up. Watch it. Tell him "No glove, no love."

7. *Don't listen to or dish gossip.* This is a hard one, I know. But some of the girls you consider to be your friends will do anything to sabotage a relationship if they're jealous of what you have. Also, nobody likes a big-mouth girl who spreads vicious rumors and lies. What you need to do is find out information on your own, and trust your own judgments.

8. *Keep your head to the sky.* Don't let anyone knock down your self-esteem. I don't know where it came from, but today, black kids seem to take special pleasure in telling someone who is smart that they're "acting white" or think they're "better than everybody else." It was never like that when my parents were growing up. That kind of thinking is for weak, shallow, stupid people. You know what you're capable of doing,

you know your potential—and if the people you hang with make fun of you for being smart or preparing for your future, you need to get rid of them immediately. Your goal in life is to do well, not play stupid so that you can hang with someone who won't even remember your name the day after you graduate from high school.

9. *To hell with smoking and drinking.* It's not cute. You get drunk, your breath stinks, your clothes get stains on them, and even though they think it's cool at the blue-light basement party, when they see you like that in the daylight, guys aren't attracted to it at all. Above all else, it's addictive and destructive. Why bother? You're not going to get anything out of it.

10. *Don't beat around the bush.* Don't send letters through your girlfriends, or ask him through his best friend's girlfriend's best friend if he likes you. Be direct; let him know you're interested and ask him if he feels the same. If he doesn't, move on to the next one. Your feelings will be hurt at first, but at least you won't spend four years like I did chasing after a guy who doesn't even know you like him—or that you even exist.

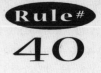
Rules for College Sistahs

Every college campus has them: the sistahs whose mission in life is to graduate with that MRS degree. Classes, GPAs, personal development, and the dean's lists take the backseat to brothers with six-figure and pro-ballplayer potential—and they work overtime to make sure that they can snatch them up before they march across that stage.

It's stupid, but true.

When I was in college, I had a few friends who didn't make a move unless it was behind the basketball team. I know a few girls who spent more than a little bit of time in the law library—and none of them were studying law. And I even knew a sistah who, in her freshman year, got pregnant within her first semester on campus by a football player she thought was going pro.

Of course, if they spent half as much time with their books as they did with those boys, they'd have it going on today for real—and every last one of them would be in an arena where the type of men they always dreamed of getting—those college-educated, professional men with big titles and even bigger money—would be ready for the taking.

Here's the scoop: College is still a very big deal in our community. It's never something that comes easy for any of us; all too often, we either come from inadequate public school systems that don't do a very good job of preparing us for the cutthroat university learning experience, or our parents can't afford the tuition. So when we get accepted to Yale and Howard and Spelman and Morehouse and Hampton University, we are still very much the first and second generations in our families to have been lucky enough to overcome the hurdles and snatch the opportunity to do that much better than our parents did. When you get there, you want to get the most out of those four years that you can.

Why squander your chance chasing after some boy who doesn't want to be chased? This is the time for you to get the best possible education you can, to make the best possible connections you can, to get that piece of paper that will lead to you getting the papers that count: the green ones. You can't do that chasing behind some man.

It's tempting, though, isn't it? We're good for throwing up those 8 to 1 sistah to brother campus ratios as reason to let him do whatever with whomever, whenever. As long as he keeps dangling that "I'm committed to you, baby" candy over our heads, we stand by him and let our grades suffer, our self-esteem drop, and our standards plummet in the hopes that we'll get the ring sometime around graduation day.

News flash: This is your time, little sistah, to get your constitution in order—to get to know yourself, to sow your "wild oats," to experiment and experience. That's, after all, what college is supposed to be about, right—learning? That doesn't just mean the kind you get in textbooks; that also means the kind you find when you take the time to get to know you.

And you can't do that if you've got your eyes trained on finding Brother Mr. Right before you complete that last semester.

Of course, it's okay to date. But play the field, girl; don't latch on to the first thing moving and then pretend like you know what you like and he's it. You're not going to know on the first try. Think about it: You don't try on one pair of shoes and walk out of the store with them, thinking you can't find anything better. If you're a smart shopper, you go to several different stores until you find the shoes you're most comfortable with and like; then you buy those. Sometimes it's the first pair you tried on; but at least you knew what else was out there before you spent all your money on the ones you ended up buying.

Well, it's the same with college guys. Why commit to the

first one, when there're so many others out there you can try on? Don't think they're not doing the same thing; I can't recall ever being around a college brother that wasn't into playing the field before he settled down with one girl—and that hardly ever happened in freshman year, or even undergrad for that matter.

Keeping yourself in check is simple. All you have to do is:

- Stay in the books—that's what you're in college for.
- Participate in extracurricular activities—like the school newspaper or the student council—to boost up that résumé and put yourself in the arena of like-minded, goal-oriented students.
- Join a sorority or sweetheart club, or create your own. It's a great outlet for creative thinking and community service—and you make a cadre of lifelong friends in the process.
- Keep yourself from committing to a brother just for the sake of committing—play the field and date a variety of brothers on and off campus to feel out what's out there and find out what you want.
- Keep yourself tight; work out, get your hair done, and pamper yourself—so that you feel good about yourself.
- Avoid following behind crowds or cliques of women who dedicate their time to following behind the potential brothers—the ones with the potential for titles and big salaries—because those brothers will automatically assume you're after them for the papers, and avoid you like the plague.

- Never, ever drink or do drugs to impress a guy or your so-called friends—because you're doing nothing but hurting yourself. Plus, it's just not cute.
- If you're having sex, always, always, ALWAYS protect yourself. You can't afford to get any diseases from unsafe sex, and you certainly can't afford to take care of any babies on that minimum-wage salary you're drawing working in the library.

Acknowledgments

All praises due to the Creator, who continues to cloak me in His unconditional love—even when I stray. I am humbled by Your power, awed by Your grace, and forever grateful for Your many blessings. Without You, I am nothing.

Thank you to my parents, James and Bettye Millner, who pegged my potential, encouraged me to push beyond it, and always cushioned my falls. I love you both so much, it hurts. Thank you, also, to my brother, Troy Millner, for your love and respect; it truly means the world to your lil' sis. And thank you, my beautiful husband, Nick Chiles, for your editing prowess, your early-morning brainstorming sessions, your crazy-ass jokes and your endless love and support. I couldn't imagine life without you.

And a bundle of "Thank Yous" to: Chikuyu and Migozo Chiles, for your well of knowledge and wisdom; Angelou Chiles Ezeilo, for being this sistah's bestest girlfriend and willing soundboard; James Ezeilo, for the slamming legal advice (You go, counselor!); Jameelah Chabwera, for letting me take those cool E-mail breaks with my new big sis; Mazi Chiles, for the cool red-pen scribbles in the margins of the hard copy and your never-ending curiosity (because of you, I can break down the meaning of the word "relationship" so that even a four-year-old can understand); and Chrisena Coleman, Tonya Fox, Laura Taylor, Jalene Auter, and Caryl Lucas for hooking a sistah up with life lessons and the companionship others only wish they had.

To my Saturday morning relief and my weekend inspirations: my students at the Legal Outreach, Inc., and Harlem Overhead, and their leaders, James O'Neal and Shawn Dove (two of the most dynamic black men I know)—thank you for keeping me grounded. You all help me focus on the more important things in life. I adore you all.

Thank you also to: Orla Healy, the best features editor a writer could ever ask for (You're brilliant!); Tom Lowe, for laying down the vision that made this all happen; Doris Cooper, for seeing that vision; and Eileen Cope, for showing me the money, and Jackie Bazan for helping me reach for it (I love you, girl!).

And I know this may look crazy, but there's a method to my madness; all my love to my two kitty cats, Stark and Jordan, for keeping Mommy company in that tiny computer room.

THE SISTAHS' RULES
money-back guarantee:

If you do not meet a good black man within one year of purchasing this book, but in no event later than January 1, 1999, get your money back. Mail the book and your receipt with a letter stating why *The Sistahs' Rules* did not work for you to:

Customer Service
William Morrow and Company, Inc.
39 Plymouth Street
P.O. Box 1269
Fairfield, N.J. 07007